FOCUS
Patient Management Exercises in Psychiatry

Editors *FOCUS* Journal

Deborah J. Hales, M.D.
Mark Hyman Rapaport, M.D.

Authors

FOCUS Patient Management Exercises in Psychiatry

B. Harrison Levine, M.D., M.P.H.
Ronald C. Albucher, M.D.

AMERICAN PSYCHIATRIC ASSOCIATION

AMERICAN PSYCHIATRIC ASSOCIATION

FOCUS Patient Management Exercises in Psychiatry

An exercise workbook covering the
ABPN outline of topics for recertification:

Anxiety Disorders
Bipolar Disorder
Child and Adolescent Psychiatry
Delirium
Gender, Race, and Culture
Major Depressive Disorder
Obsessive-Compulsive Disorder
Panic Disorder
Personality Disorders
Psychopharmacology
Psychotherapy
Schizophrenia
Sleep, Sex, and Eating Disorders
Substance Abuse

B. Harrison Levine, M.D., M.P.H.

Ronald C. Albucher, M.D.

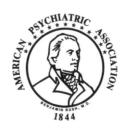

Manufactured in the United States of America on acid-free paper

American Psychiatric Association
1000 Wilson Boulevard
Arlington, VA 22209-3901
www.psych.org

Library of Congress Cataloging-in-Publication Data
A CIP record is available from the Library of Congress.

British Library Cataloguing in Publication Data
A CIP record is available from the British Library.

Table of Contents

FOCUS Patient Management Exercises in Psychiatry

FOCUS Patient Management Exercises in Psychiatry is a practical and accessible self-study workbook designed for practicing psychiatrists. Physicians who complete the exercises in this workbook can improve their clinical decision making, advance their communication and diagnostic abilities, evaluate their knowledge and clinical skills, learn leading-edge clinical information, and most importantly, improve patient care.

Sixteen clinical vignettes are presented in the following topic areas:

Anxiety Disorders
Bipolar Disorder
Child and Adolescent Psychiatry
Delirium
Gender, Race, and Culture
Major Depressive Disorder
Obsessive-Compulsive Disorder

Panic Disorder
Personality Disorders
Psychopharmacology
Psychotherapy
Schizophrenia
Sleep, Sex, and Eating Disorders
Substance Abuse

These exercises are designed to test the psychiatrist's clinical considerations beyond the typical multiple-choice testing approach. They describe diagnostic and therapeutic questions in a clinical narrative that follows a patient through the passage of time. Each vignette attempts to closely resemble actual patient presentations. Physicians often confront contradictory or confusing constellations of symptoms, and patients may introduce new and critical information that was unexpected by the physician. These clinical vignettes can help refine diagnostic skills and facilitate sharpening practitioners' clinical decision making.

This book is meant to be used in a program of continuous professional development. It will help psychiatrists assess their processes of evaluation, diagnosis, and clinical management. These exercises may also be useful in preparing for board-type examinations, and they have been found to promote discussion and learning for individuals of various levels of experience, ranging from seasoned clinicians to psychiatric residents. The vignettes that follow promote competence in clinical decision making and patient care. The case-based, problem-oriented approach is a valuable and stimulating learning tool for both trainees and established practitioners.

Each vignette places the reader in a clinical situation with a specific patient and asks for clinical judgments that psychiatrists make regularly in practice. Cases are presented with an emphasis on decisions that are made in the course of actual patient care. The patient is introduced, and at selected decision points, the task is to choose a practice option appropriate for that patient at that point in time. Each case highlights different key clinical concepts that can be incorporated into one's practice. As one works through the exercises, one can score in real time one's choices related to diagnosis, communication, level of care, type of treatment, and potential complications—virtually everything encountered in a clinical setting. This can enhance the integration of new knowledge by presenting it in a clinically relevant fashion.

Up to 32 hours of AMA PRA category 1 credits™ are available for completing the patient management exercises in this workbook. Work is completed independently in the book and the participant self-scores the results. A score of 60% or higher is required to earn CME credit. Credit is awarded online at www.apaeducation.org.

We hope that you will find *FOCUS Patient Management Exercises in Psychiatry* to be a clinically useful educational activity.

B. Harrison Levine, M.D., M.P.H.

Ronald C. Albucher, M.D.

FOCUS Patient Management Exercises in Psychiatry

HOW TO USE THIS BOOK

The case vignettes for each of the 16 exercises place the reader in clinical situations at different decision points. One or more choices may be correct, and choices should be made on the basis of clinical knowledge and the history of the patient provided. Read all the options for each question before making a selection. You are given points on a graded scale for the best possible answer(s) (in order of importance), and points are deducted for answers that would result in a poor outcome or a delay in arriving at the right answer. Options with little or no impact on the patient receive zero points. On questions that focus on a differential diagnosis, bonus points are awarded for selecting the most likely diagnosis as your first choice. At the end of the exercise, add up the points to obtain a total score and rationale. Key clinical concepts, summarizing the important clinical learning objectives, are included at the end of each exercise.

Program release date: May 2011

Program end date: May 2014

Accreditation: The American Psychiatric Association is accredited by the Accreditation Council for Continuing Medical Education (ACCME) to provide continuing medical education for physicians.

*The American Psychiatric Association designates this enduring material for a maximum of **32** AMA PRA category 1 credits.™ Physicians should claim only the credit commensurate with the extent of their participation in the activity.*

Educational Objectives

By completing the exercises in this workbook physicians will:

- Improve clinical decision making and patient care
- Advance their communication, diagnostic, and treatment skills
- Evaluate their knowledge and clinical skills

HOW TO EARN CME CREDIT

To earn AMA PRA category 1 credit,™ the total score for each exercise should be 60% of the ideal score (or higher). All work is done in the workbook, but the CME credits are awarded online. To claim credit and receive your certificate, go to www.apaeducation.org and click the link "***Enter CME Code for Credit***" in the left navigation menu under Books and Journals. Log in using your username and password. If you don't have a username and password, please click the link to create a new account. After you log in, enter the CME Code on the scratch-off sticker on **the inside back cover** of your book and click "Proceed to Course Enrollment." Confirm that the title displayed is correct – select OK. The course will appear on your Student Home page. Launch the course to complete the evaluation and claim credit. Once the course is completed, you will be able to print your certificate from the My Transcript section.

Target Audience: General psychiatrists, psychiatrists in clinical practice; psychiatric residents and fellows; medical students interested in psychiatry; physicians who wish to improve their knowledge of clinical psychiatry and patient care.

Author Affiliation and Disclosure of Financial Interests or Other Affiliations with Commercial Organizations

Ronald C. Albucher, M.D.

Clinical Associate Professor of Psychiatry, Stanford University and Director of Stanford's Counseling and Psychological Services Center

Dr. Albucher reports no competing interests.

B. Harrison Levine, M.D., M.P.H.

Associate Professor, Division of Child and Adolescent Psychiatry, University of Colorado Health Sciences Center

Dr. Levine reports no competing interests.

CME Program Planners Affiliation and Disclosure of Financial Interests or Other Affiliations with Commercial Organizations

Deborah J. Hales, M.D.

Director, American Psychiatric Association Division of Education, Co-Editor *FOCUS: The Journal of Lifelong Learning in Psychiatry*

Dr. Hales reports no competing interests.

Mark Hyman Rapaport, M.D.

Chairman, Department of Psychiatry, Cedars-Sinai Medical Center, Co-Editor *FOCUS: The Journal of Lifelong Learning in Psychiatry*

Consultant: Affectis, Astellas, Brain Cells Inc., Johnson & Johnson, Methylation, PAX, Pfizer, Quintiles; *Grant/Research Support:* NCCAM, NIMH.

Hardware/Software

This activity takes place both in the workbook and online; no special software other than a standard web browser is needed.

For questions about *FOCUS Patient Management Exercises in Psychiatry* contact:

American Psychiatric Association
Dept. of CME
1000 Wilson Blvd. Suite 1825
Arlington, VA 22209
703/907-8631
educme@psych.org

You Are Touching the Door

Vignette part 1

You are an emergency room psychiatrist. A young man, 18 years of age, is brought in by ambulance after he "destroyed" the trailer in which he and his mother had been living. The precipitant is not clear. The young man's mother accompanied him to the psychiatric emergency room. Two nurses and an emergency room technician help the Emergency Medical Services (EMS) team to transfer the patient from the ambulance to a hospital gurney where he is placed in four-point restraints by three hospital security officers owing to his continuing aggressive and assaultive behavior. With a great deal of difficulty you check the patient's vital signs (heart rate 120 beats per minute, blood pressure 180/85 mm Hg, respiratory rate 20, and temperature 98.4°F) and examine the patient grossly for any obvious signs of trauma or injury. He is disheveled, malodorous, and appears to have been wearing the same torn jeans and filthy T-shirt for some time. He is average height and weight for his age but appears older given his unkempt appearance. You attempt to speak with him, but he refuses to answer you, and you notice his hands and teeth are clenched tightly. For the most part, he stares at the ceiling, but occasionally his eyes dart around as if someone else is talking to him.

The EMS team reports that he was silent after an initial struggle with police to remove him from his home. His mother tells you he started behaving "strangely" approximately 3 months ago, insisting that their trailer was under surveillance and there were men following him whom he did not know, but he was sure they were from the government and meant to harm him. He stopped leaving the trailer and quit taking showers. He stayed up all night watching the TV without the sound on and slept most of the day. Two weeks ago he began removing some of the plumbing in the trailer because he said it was "bugged." The patient's mother

works at a paper mill; she said that her son started calling her cell phone up to 10 times a day to be sure she was "safe."

While you are attempting to get history from the patient's mother he begins to yell obscenities at a nurse who is standing nearby. The mother denies his taking any medications of any sort. She tells you he has been smoking her cigarettes because "he has been running out of his more and more" and this bothers her because "smokes are so expensive now. I cannot afford to buy so many." She is not sure if he uses street drugs, but he does not drink alcohol at home where he spends most of his time. He has no general medical problems. During this interview, the patient's agitation is escalating. You see him struggling with the leather restraints until he manages to free his right leg. He begins kicking the wall beside the gurney. Several people in the waiting room watch the proceedings anxiously.

Decision Point A

Given what you know about the patient and the behaviors you are witnessing, what is the most appropriate first step you should take in managing this patient? Points awarded for correct and incorrect answers are scaled from best (+5) to unhelpful but not harmful (0) to dangerous (−5).

A1. _____ Remove the remaining restraints yourself as these are obviously the cause of his worsening agitation. Triage him as the most urgent case in the emergency room and ask him to accompany you into the closest open interview room.

A2. _____ Ask the security officers to remove the remaining restraints as these are obviously the cause of his worsening agitation. Triage him as the most urgent case in the emergency room and ask him to accompany you into the closest open interview room.

A3. _____ Ask the security officers to restrain the patient's freed leg and then wheel him to the isolation room. Once he is safely restrained and inside the room, ask everyone to leave the patient alone and close the door. Continue your interview with the patient's mother.

A4. _____ Ask the security officers to restrain the patient's freed leg and then wheel him to the isolation room. Try to calm the patient by speaking to him in a calm voice. If this is unsuccessful, ask the patient if he is willing to take an oral medication that will help him relax. Tell him if he does not take the oral medication you will have to give him an injection of medicine that will help him relax. This patient is severely agitated, so medications must be delivered promptly.

A5. _____ Ask the security officers to restrain the patient's freed leg and then wheel him to the isolation room. Give him an injection of haloperidol 5 mg, lorazepam 2 mg, and benztropine 1 mg. Wait 15–20 minutes for the medications to take effect. If he is still combative, give another identical injection.

VIGNETTE PART 2

The patient calms down considerably after he agreed to take a total of olanzapine (orally disintegrating tablet) 10 mg, given in 5-mg doses 1 hour apart. He is no longer in restraints but prefers to remain in the isolation room where he is resting on the gurney. The door to the isolation room is kept open, and a nurse is sitting in a chair just outside the doorway. He asks to speak with you. He tells you that he knows his trailer is bugged by the FBI and the CIA because, "I know too much. They have been watching me and my mother." He expresses worry that the FBI or the CIA plans to kidnap his mother to "make me talk." This is why he has been calling her. "But she does not get it. She does not get it. She does not get it. I have to get it."

He denies feeling sad or hopeless but endorses feeling helpless to stop the government agencies from "harassing us." He has thought about killing himself in the past but denies current suicidal thoughts. The last time he was suicidal was approximately 1 month ago. You decide to make a gentle assumption that he is hearing voices and ask, "What are they telling you?" He closes his eyes and says, "It is always about how I need to kill myself or kill my mother because that is what the government wants. That is how I knew I had to get rid of the pipes." He thought about killing his mother to save her from the FBI and the CIA, but then decided against that because "Then they've got me, they've got me, they get me, they get me. It is me, it is me, it is me, it is me." He tells you he

has found "poison" in some of the food his mother has brought home for him to eat. Sometimes he only eats potato chips for days, which he asserts cannot be poisoned because they are "crispy."

He said he lost his job at a fast-food restaurant two months ago because "They did not get it, did not get it, they did not get it. It is me." He quit high school at the beginning of 11th grade. He does not see friends anymore because he is convinced they have been compromised by the government and are spying on him. "I do see Nick every day, though. He lives two rows over. We smoke weed together." Then he adds, "Don't tell my mother." He then turns away on the gurney and seems to sleep.

You speak with his mother. She tells you that he used to be a B student until the end of 10th grade when his grades started to deteriorate. He worked during that summer at a fast-food restaurant and seemed to do well, although he had a few bouts of feeling low. He was never violent or aggressive. At some point early in 11th grade he got into a physical altercation with another student and threatened to kill him. He was taken from school by ambulance to your psychiatric emergency room, evaluated, found to be upset but not a danger to anyone or to himself, and was discharged to follow-up at an outpatient child and adolescent psychiatric clinic connected to your hospital. His mother said he never went to any appointments because he insisted, "I'm not crazy. You are." He had never taken any psychiatric medications, was never previously hospitalized for psychiatric reasons, and, although he was staying home more and more, his mother never felt the need to pressure her son into treatment. "I have to work to support us," she tells you. "I cannot keep track of everything."

DECISION POINT B

Given what you know about this patient so far, what would be your next steps in assessing the patient? Points awarded for correct and incorrect answers are scaled from best (+5) to unhelpful but not harmful (0) to dangerous (−5).

B1. _____ The patient is clearly schizophrenic and needs to be taking antipsychotic medications. Arrange with his mother for the patient to be seen in your outpatient department, and as soon as the patient is stable, discharge him home to his mother's care.

B2. _____ The patient is clearly schizophrenic and needs to be taking antipsychotic medications. Given the good response from olanzapine, give the mother a prescription for a month's supply of olanzapine 10 mg PO at bedtime, arrange the first available appointment at your outpatient department which is in 5 days, and explain to her that she should bring him back to the psychiatric emergency room if he again decompensates.

B3. _____ Order the following laboratory values and studies: rheumatoid factor, antinuclear antibodies, erythrocyte sedimentation rate, vitamin B_{12}, folate, Lyme disease titer, complete blood count with differential, Chem-7, liver function tests, thyroid-stimulating hormone, urinalysis, urine toxicology screen, computed tomographic (CT) scan of the head without contrast, and an electrocardiogram (ECG). Obtain further history, especially a family history of psychiatric illness.

B4. _____ If you are able to rule out a general medical cause to his psychosis, start aripiprazole 5 mg PO treat-

ment for the patient at bedtime and discharge to the care of his mother. Schedule the first available appointment at your outpatient department which is in 5 days and explain to her that she should bring him back to the psychiatric emergency room if he again decompensates.

B5. _____ Order the laboratory values and studies in answer B3 and then admit the patient to an adolescent inpatient unit for further evaluation and safety.

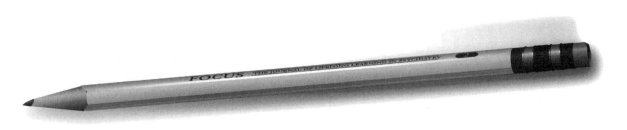

DECISION POINT C

Given what you know about this patient, what is your differential diagnosis? Points are given for correct answers, and negative points for incorrect answers.

AXIS I:	
AXIS II:	

VIGNETTE PART 3

Once it was determined the patient did not have an underlying organic cause to his psychiatric symptoms, he was hospitalized in an adolescent in-patient unit. His urine toxicology screen was negative for substances, including cannabis. He is started on risperidone, which is quickly titrated to 3mg BID over the course of 2 weeks with good results. The patient no longer appears agitated, is sleeping well, is eating all of his meals, and speaks freely with you. However, he is still mostly isolative on the unit, preferring to listen to music through headphones or watch TV with some peers. He tells you that he has gone without sleep for 2–3 days at a time, but feels exhausted all day when he is unable to sleep. He admits he had been hearing a voice in his head telling him what he was doing as he did it, such as "you are now walking," or "you are touching the door." He also heard two different voices talking to him or about him, sometimes saying "I should kill myself," or "I have to kill my mother." He still thinks you are recording him, but he tells you, "if that is what you gotta do, then that is what you gotta do." He no longer believes the food in the unit

is poisoned, although he does recall thinking that before. He has poor recollection of the details surrounding his admission to the hospital.

He says he does not have any hobbies other than "smoking cigarettes" and listening to music. Until recently, however, he typically would go outside and walk and visit his neighbor, and previously he spent a great deal of time doing schoolwork. He says he usually has good energy, but finds it difficult to concentrate more and more. "It did not used to be like that," he tells you. His appetite now is strong, and he believes it is because of the medication.

Further history revealed that his mother was in treatment for depression, his biological father and paternal uncle both suffered from schizophrenia, and he had a paternal great aunt who lived in a state psychiatric hospital for many years but died before the patient was born. According to the patient's mother, she noticed that her son was "a little slow to speak," a little clumsy, and did not socialize very well with age-appropriate peers as he grew up. Her pediatrician told her he was within the normal range of development and an evaluation of developmental delays was not pursued. He never had a girlfriend, nor did he seem particularly interested in romantic pursuits. By 11th grade, however, he began to isolate more, he seemed outwardly depressed, he stopped doing much of his homework, and his grades began to slide. Three months into the school year, 4 months before this emergency room visit, the patient quit school and refused to leave the trailer except to visit a neighbor where he allegedly smoked marijuana, and his mother noted that she often caught him talking to himself. At first, she said, he would look frightened if she found him speaking out loud to himself, as if he were in trouble. Eventually, he did not seem to care if he was talking to himself in front of her. She never understood what he was talking about, but she recalls he was anxious and nervous, looking around the trailer as if he were being watched. "Then he started telling me these crazy things about the government spying on us, that our trailer was bugged."

They began to argue more. She tried to stop him from removing wiring, dismantling a lamp, opening up the back of the TV, and other "odd behaviors," but he would "fly into a rage at me" and threaten to hit her "for my own good." He would scream loudly to leave him alone. Over the past 3 weeks she often found him sobbing in his room and unable to tell her why except for repeating, "Why can't I just die?" Their fights quickly intensified both verbally and physically. The patient shoved his mother a couple of times but never hit her. She said she was now fearful he would harm her. He also began threatening to kill himself with a gun. They did not own a gun, but she thought the neighbor might own one.

DECISION POINT D

From what you have learned about the patient, what is the most important factor you should explore next? Points awarded for correct and incorrect answers are scaled from best (+5) to unhelpful but not harmful (0) to dangerous (−5).

D1. _____ Obtain as much collateral information as is possible, from the mother, other doctors, teachers, and even friends.

D2. _____ Call the police to investigate the patient's neighbor who may be supplying the patient with marijuana.

D3. _____ Evaluate the mother for psychiatric illness and recommend treatment.

D4. _____ Evaluate the patient's suicidal and homicidal risks. Provide education to the patient's mother about how to "sterilize" her home from easy methods of self-harm or suicide, such as locking away pills, knives, and removing any firearms from the home.

D5. _____ Contact the FBI and the CIA and determine whether your patient is actually the subject of an inquiry or investigation.

DECISION POINT E

Which of the following features of schizophrenia represent good or bad prognoses? Answer by checking the correct box. +2 points are given for correct answers, −2 points for incorrect answers.

Feature	Good Prognosis	Bad Prognosis
E1. Younger onset		
E2. Good premorbid interpersonal function		
E3. Poor social supports		
E4. Short active psychotic phase		
E5. Family history of schizophrenia		
E6. Family history of mood disorders		
E7. Multiple relapses		
E8. Insidious onset		
E9. Prolonged active psychotic phase		
E10. Prominent positive symptoms		

ANSWERS: SCORING, RELATIVE WEIGHTS, AND COMMENTS

DECISION POINT A

Generally, management of an acutely agitated patient in the emergency setting should begin with attempts to deescalate the patient using nonpharmacological methods. The clinician should begin by making sure both he or she and the patient have easy access to an escape route from this engagement. Additionally, by speaking in a nonconfrontational, soft, friendly tone, exhibiting body language that is nonthreatening, avoiding direct eye contact, and maintaining a safe distance to avoid encroachment upon the patient's personal space have been shown as preventative against provoking stress and anxiety in the patient. Immediate assessment of suicidal and/or homicidal ideation should be performed. If these measures are sufficient, the use of chemical or physical restraints may be avoided. Otherwise, attempts to use pharmacological interventions should be tried. It may become necessary to physically restrain the patient and then use medications to calm the patient. Prolonged use of physical restraints while a patient struggles can lead to unintentional self-harm, hyperkalemia, rhabdomyolysis, and cardiac arrest, and subsequently the use of medications can reduce these risks.

If a patient is physically restrained, there must be regular and frequent evaluation of the patient's cardiovascular and neurological status and examination of the patient's extremities, respiration, and hemodynamics. These assessments should be clearly documented, along with the reason for the restraint procedure(s), or continuation of the restraint procedure(s).

A1. _____ −5 The first step in managing an acutely agitated patient is for staff to attempt to calm the patient by talking to him or her. If this is not possible, staff who are trained in safe restraint procedures should restrain the patient in a way that minimizes risk of harm to the patient or to staff. Removing restraints for an acutely agitated patient, especially in an emergency room waiting area, is dangerous as the patient is probably frightened and confused, and there is a high likelihood of his or her causing harm to themselves or to others. You should never place yourself or anyone else in a closed room with an acutely agitated and possibly psychotic patient who is not medicated or restrained.

A2. _____ −5 It is an appropriate practice to ask specially trained staff (here, the security officers) to apply restraints. Restraining the freed leg is important as this patient is using his leg in such a way that he might hurt himself or others. However, despite finding the most appropriate person to remove restraints, this particular patient is currently too dangerous in his current state and the restraints should not be removed. Removing him from the common area of the emergency

room will keep others safe and not contribute to the escalation of other waiting patient's symptoms. Keeping the patient in a closed room without medications or restraints may help calm the patient, but the room should not have furniture or fixtures that can be used by the patient to harm himself or others. As soon as it is possible, medications should be used to help calm the patient so that the restraints may be removed. In addition, the patient should be monitored either by close-circuit TV if available to the emergency room or by frequent 15-minute checks by staff, which is a Joint Commission on Accreditation of Healthcare Organizations and ethical "must."

A3. _____ −5 Leaving the patient alone in restraints when he is clearly in a severely agitated state without medications is not likely to relieve his symptoms and could worsen his symptoms. Use of trained staff to manipulate restraints is appropriate, especially because this patient may hurt himself or others. Removing him from the common area of the emergency room will keep others safe and not contribute to the escalation of other, waiting patient's symptoms. First attempting to calm the patient with a soft voice can often deescalate an agitated patient and avoid the need for more aggressive measures. If this is not possible, the use of restraints should be used to help the patient safely receive a short-acting neuroleptic with or without an anxiolytic. Benztropine, an anticholinergic medication, is often used in combination with first-generation neuroleptics to reduce the risk of drug-induced extrapyramidal movements, rigidity, tremor, and gait disturbances

A4. _____ +5 Because of the severity of this particular patient's agitation, his symptoms should be treated with medications as quickly as possible to avoid any potential harm he might cause himself or others, despite the restraints. It is preferable to use a second-generation neuroleptic such as risperidone or olanzapine, both of which come in rapidly dissolving tablets to minimize the potential for "cheeking" or spitting out the medication. In a young male patient, the atypical agents are preferred over first-generation neuroleptics such as haloperidol because the latter is associated with a higher risk of drug-induced extrapyramidal movements, rigidity, tremor, and gait disturbances, or the more serious and life-threatening neuroleptic malignant syndrome. If the patient is unable to take the tablet or refuses, most states allow for emergency administration of an injectable parenteral neuroleptic such as the first generation neuroleptic haloperidol or second-generation neuroleptics such as ziprasidone and olanzapine. The choice of whether to use first or second-generation neuroleptics, benzodiazepines, or a combination of the two should be considered on a case-to-case basis, taking into account the patient's previous or current psychiatric medications, his or her response to those medications, and his or her age, sex, general medical comorbidities, or risk factors.

A5. ____ −3 In practice, especially in the emergency setting with an acutely agitated, possibly psychotic patient, there is an urgency to reduce potential for harm to the patient or to others. Waiting 15–20 minutes for the medications to take effect may or may not be enough time. Generally, the purpose of using medications is to calm the patient and reduce the symptoms but not to sedate the patient. The overarching principle is maintaining patient and staff safety. However, the use of multiple medications, including an atypical antipsychotic in a male patient is potentially dangerous.

DECISION POINT B

Generally, when one evaluates a patient in an acute psychotic state, it is very important to obtain as much collateral information as possible as this patient is unlikely to give a coherent or accurate history. The possible etiologies of psychosis are numerous and the clinician should begin with a general medical and psychiatric examination, including patient and family history, level of premorbid functioning, chronology, intensity of symptoms, general medical history, substance use history.

B1. ____ −5 The patient may appear to be schizophrenic; however, you cannot yet make this diagnosis without first ruling out any general medical causes of his psychosis. Additionally, he has demonstrated that he is a danger to himself and to his mother. His symptoms have been worsening over 3 months, but you have been given clues that a prodrome of illness may have begun approximately 2 years ago. This patient should be hospitalized for further evaluation, stabilization, safety, and treatment.

B2. ____ −3 See B1. Additionally, the patient's response to olanzapine (orally disintegrating tablet) 10 mg comprised primarily a reduction of his behavioral dyscontrol and moderate organization of his thought process. However, he is still in thought-disordered and perseverating phrases, demonstrating some looseness of associations, and delusions of surveillance, paranoia, and persecution. As stated above in B1, this patient should be hospitalized for further evaluation, stabilization, safety, and treatment.

B3. ____ +5 There are many medical and neurological conditions that can present with psychosis. Medical conditions associated with psychosis include neurological, infectious, metabolic, oncological, and immunological processes, as well as alcohol and drug intoxication or withdrawal and vitamin deficiency. Among the most common presentations of such changes in mental status include neurological disorders including meningitis, encephalitis, cerebrovascular accidents, subarachnoid hemorrhages, and subdural hematoma. Other, less common neurological causes of psychosis include brain tumors, metastases to the central nervous system, seizure disorders, or a neurodegenerative disease (especially with young children). Metabolic disorders include myxedema, thyrotoxicosis, Cushing's disease, and less commonly diabetes. The anoxia from pulmonary disease can present with psychotic-like symptoms. Other considerations include porphyria or Wilson's disease, both of which may present first with psychiatric symptoms before the physical etiology becomes clear. Lupus erythematosus can cause an "organic" psychosis, or the treatment for lupus, corticosteroids, can also cause psychosis. Deficiencies in nicotinic acid or thiamine as well as lead intoxication can cause psychotic symptoms. Medications the patient may be taking, either prescription or street drugs, can also cause psychotic symptoms. Withdrawal symptoms from some of these medications or drugs can also present as psychosis. In this latter category, urine toxicology screening is necessary as these patients are often unable or unwilling to reveal whether they ingested medications or street drugs.

There are no official guidelines for which laboratory values or studies to order. It has become commonplace for psychiatrists minimally to order a complete blood count with differential, liver function tests, thyroid-stimulating hormone, urinalysis, and urine toxicology screen for most psychiatric patients to help rule out organic causes of psychiatric symptoms or to check organ function if medications are to be used. Additionally, an ECG has become especially important as many of the neuroleptics (as well as other classes of psychoactive medications) affect cardiac conduction, often by widening QTc intervals. In younger, healthy patients with no known history of heart disease, obtaining an ECG is not as important as initially thought. However, there is no consensus concerning the other laboratory values and studies and many clinicians choose to err on the side of safety. Others believe that the clinical and epidemiological picture should direct which laboratory values and studies should be ordered. For example, if this patient demonstrated focal neurological signs or a history of head trauma, a CT scan of the head without contrast would be indicated. Many neurologists would prefer a magnetic resonance imaging scan to evaluate more temporally distant insults as well. Even though the yield for a positive result is quite low, most clinicians prefer to rule out a general medical cause to the symptoms no matter the cost because the results affect treatment decisions.

B4. _____ −5 Despite the reasonable approach of first eliminating organic causes to the patient's symptoms, he should not be discharged but hospitalized for the same reasons given in answers B1 and B2.

B5. _____ +5 Most hospitals insist upon many of these studies before they will accept a patient to their inpatient unit. Additionally, before the patient leaves the emergency department, "organic" causes should be ruled out to avoid hospitalizing the patient in a psychiatric unit when a medical unit is necessary to further evaluate and treat medical illness with psychiatric symptoms.

DECISION POINT C

Axis I:	(−2) Brief Psychotic Disorder; (+2) Schizophreniform Disorder; (+2) Rule out Schizophrenia; (+2) Rule out Schizoaffective Disorder; (−2) Delusional Disorder; (+1) Rule out Major Depressive Disorder with Psychotic Features; (−2) Rule out Bipolar Disorder with Psychotic Features; (−2) Delirium; (−2) Dementia; (+1 pt) Rule out substance-induced psychotic disorder; (−2) Psychosis secondary to a general medical condition
Axis II:	(−2) Rule out Schizoid Personality Disorder; (−2) Rule out Schizotypal Personality Disorder; (−2) Rule out Borderline Personality Disorder

Diagnostic criteria for schizophrenia according to DSM-IV-TR are shown in Table 1.

Brief Psychotic Disorder (−2). This patient had symptoms greater than 1 month in duration. For this diagnosis, the symptoms must last from 1 day to 1 month.

Schizophreniform Disorder (+2). We are told the patient's symptoms worsened over the previous 3 months. There may have been prodromal symptoms lasting longer, especially given the patient's quitting school 4 months earlier. Aggressive behavior is associated with schizophrenia, although violence is not. Risk factors for aggression in schizophrenia are male gender; being poor, unskilled, uneducated, or unmarried; and having a history of prior arrests or a prior history of violence. This risk increases with comorbid alcohol or substance abuse, antisocial personality, or neurological impairment. Given the unreliability of the patient's history and mother's minimizing of previous symptoms, we cannot be certain the symptoms have been present for more than 6 months. Until we know better, or until more time has passed, the patient can safely be diagnosed with schizophreniform disorder. It should be noted, however, that approximately two-thirds of patients will proceed to schizophrenia or schizoaffective disorder.

Rule out Schizophrenia (+2). The patient demonstrates two symptoms from Criterion A, including the voice of a running commentary and two voices conversing with each other. The caveats to this diagnosis are establishing criteria C through F. The time frame for the absolute length of his illness is difficult to determine given that the patient is a poor historian and his mother may have minimized his symptoms. The normal physical examination and normal results for laboratory values and studies make it unlikely that this patient has a general medical condition that could be causing the symptoms. The role of substance abuse (marijuana) was not ruled out, and further testing is necessary to absolutely rule out a pervasive developmental disorder. The patient did demonstrate "soft" neurological signs since he was a baby and was somewhat socially challenged, although he did manage to do very well in mainstream education until his symptoms worsened in 11th grade. Although it seems quite likely that this is the patient's primary diagnosis, clinicians should be careful when labeling a patient, especially an adolescent, with a diagnosis such as schizophrenia. If incorrect, this diagnosis could adversely affect the patient's ability to recover because of the

---

Table 1. DIAGNOSTIC CRITERIA FOR SCHIZOPHRENIA

A. *Characteristic symptoms:* Two (or more) of the following, each present for a significant portion of time during a 1-month period (or less if successfully treated):

  1. delusions

  2. hallucinations

  3. disorganized speech (e.g., frequent derailment or incoherence)

  4. grossly disorganized or catatonic behavior

Note: Only one Criterion A symptom is required if delusions are bizarre or hallucinations consist of a voice keeping up a running commentary on the person's behavior or thoughts, or two or more voices conversing with each other.

B. *Social/occupational dysfunction:* For a significant portion of the time since the onset of the disturbance, one or more major areas of functioning such as work, interpersonal relations, or self-care are markedly below the level achieved prior to the onset (or when the onset is in childhood or adolescence, failure to achieve expected level of interpersonal, academic, or occupational achievement).

C. *Duration:* Continuous signs of the disturbance persist for at least 6 months. This 6-month period must include at least 1 month of symptoms (or less if successfully treated) that meet Criterion A (i.e., active-phase symptoms) and may include periods of prodromal or residual symptoms. During these prodromal or residual periods, the signs of the disturbance may be manifested by only negative symptoms or two or more symptoms listed in Criterion A present in an attenuated form (e.g., odd beliefs, unusual perceptual experiences).

D. *Schizoaffective and Mood Disorder exclusion:* Schizoaffective Disorder and Mood Disorder With Psychotic Features have been ruled out because either (1) no Major Depressive, Manic, or Mixed Episodes have occurred concurrently with the active-phase symptoms; or (2) if mood episodes have occurred during active-phase symptoms, their total duration has been brief relative to the duration of the active and residual periods.

E. *Substance/general medical condition exclusion:* The disturbance is not due to the direct physiological effects of a substance (e.g., a drug of abuse, a medication) or a general medical condition.

F. *Relationship to a Pervasive Developmental Disorder:* If there is a history of Autistic Disorder or another Pervasive Developmental Disorder, the additional diagnosis of Schizophrenia is made only if prominent delusions or hallucinations are also present for at least a month (or less if successfully treated)

Reprinted from Diagnostic and Statistical Manual of Mental Disorders, 4th Edition, Text Revision. Copyright © 2000. American Psychiatric Association Used with Permission.

---

stigma of this illness, both from the patient's perspective and from that of others who may learn of this patient's diagnosis. It will also affect future treatment considerations.

Rule out Schizoaffective Disorder (+2). This disorder occurs at approximately 10% the rate of schizophrenia and can be distinguished by the presence of a mood disorder, such as major depression and/or mania during a significant portion of the illness. However, there must be at least 2 weeks of psychotic symptoms in the absence of major mood symptoms to meet the criteria for schizoaffective disorder. This patient may have experienced major mood symptoms, or his insomnia could have been the result of not being able to sleep because of symptoms related to psychosis, such as voices, paranoid ideation, or other anxiety-provoking disturbances of thought content or form. Patients with schizophrenia often have a mood disturbance, such as depression, but it is not typically a major mood disturbance. Until a more clear history is determined, this illness remains a rule-out.

Delusional Disorder (−2). The patient's symptoms point more towards a schizophreniform disorder or schizophrenia than for a delusional disorder, which by criterion B of delusional disorder disqualifies this diagnosis. Additionally, the patient's delusions are quite bizarre. For a delusional disorder they should be non-bizarre.

Rule out Major Depressive Disorder with Psychotic Features (+1). The patient is described by his mother as appearing depressed, tearful for the past 3 weeks, voicing suicidal ideation, and isolating, with the patient endorsing difficulty concentrating. The patient's psychotic symptoms have been described in detail. He may have a major depressive disorder with psychotic features or perhaps a depressive disorder, but his primary diagnosis is more likely a psychotic disorder. The range of patients with schizophrenia who experience depressive symptoms ranges from 7% to 75%.

Rule out Bipolar Disorder with Psychotic Features (−2). The patient does not endorse classic or atypical symptoms of mania. His insomnia is more likely due to a depression or psychotic symptoms. The patient exhibits classic Schneiderian psychotic symptoms, including hearing a voice that offers a running commentary about his actions and two voices that speak either to him or to each other about him.

Delirium (−2). The patient was evaluated for general medical causes of his changed mental status and the findings were negative. He had no evidence of waxing or waning consciousness, and no evidence of sudden onset of symptoms.

Dementia (−2). Given the patient's age and normal physical findings, normal laboratory values and imaging studies, this diagnosis is highly unlikely.

Rule Out Substance-Induced Psychotic Disorder (+1). Results of the patient's urine toxicology screen was negative, despite his assertion that he regularly smokes "weed." Tetrahydrocannabinol has a very long half-life in the human body and can be detected up to 1 month or more after last use of the substance, especially if used regularly. Although it is highly unlikely that his symptoms are the result of current use of substances, the positive threshold of the urine toxicology screen may be too high for the amount the patient actually smoked, his illness may have begun as a result of his abuse of substances, or he may be using substances that are not readily discernible with a standard six-substance urine toxicology screen. There is also the possibility of a false-negative result. Care should be given to explore the patient's actual use of substances and alcohol, given his assertion that he does use marijuana regularly.

Psychosis Secondary to a General Medical Condition (−2). The patient has been examined and is physically healthy.

Schizoid Personality Disorder (−2). This patient probably has an axis I diagnosis, not a personality disorder. There was a prodrome to his illness and then a worsening of psychotic symptoms. His premorbid functioning was within the normal range.

Schizotypal Personality Disorder (−2). There is no pervasive pattern of social and interpersonal deficits. He does have many of the symptoms of a schizotypal personality disorder, such as odd beliefs, audio hallucinations, paranoid ideation, odd behaviors, and a lack of close friends. However, his symptoms are better accounted for by an axis I diagnosis.

Borderline Personality Disorder (−2). As above, there is no pervasive pattern of instability of interpersonal relationships, self-image, and affects. His symptoms are better accounted for by an axis I diagnosis.

DECISION POINT D

D1. _____ +3 This is a necessary step in evaluating any patient. In a patient with suspected schizophrenia, there is an assumption that the patient may be thought disordered and therefore unable to provide a cogent, accurate history. Additionally, this is a young patient who is unlikely to know his own developmental history, academic history, general medical history, or behavioral history as witnessed by the various individuals who know him.

D2. _____ −5 Your job is not to be a police detective, but the patient's doctor. Although it would be infor-mative to know more information about the patient's alleged marijuana abuse, the neighbor may have nothing to do with the situation. It is certainly not your responsibility to investigate a theoretical criminal matter.

D3. _____ +1 The mother is not your patient. While speaking with her, you can ask about her own condition in terms of family psychiatric history or to provide support if she needs it. If she wants an evaluation and she does not have a psychiatrist or other clinician working with her, or if she wants a new clinician, you can certainly provide referrals. However, she has not presented to your psychiatric emergency room for herself, but brought in her son. She has not indicated to you that she is in any danger to herself or to others, so there is no need to treat her as a patient. It is good practice, however, to be empathetic to her concerns, listen carefully, and develop a good rapport as you will want her to be actively involved and appropriately educated on the treatment of her son.

D4. _____ +5 This patient has expressed suicidal ideation in the past and has mentioned the use of a gun to kill himself. As many as 30% of schizophrenic patients attempt suicide and between 4 and 10% complete suicide. Suicidal behavior is prevalent in between 20 and 40% of schizophrenic patients. In this case, the patient experienced command auitory hallucinations, which have been found to increase the risk of suicide. The patient has also threatened his mother's life. It should be noted, however, that patients with schizophrenia do not generally demonstrate a higher risk for homicide than individuals within the general population.

D5. _____ −5 Although it may be true that some people are being pursued by the FBI or the CIA, this is clearly not the case in this patient's presentation. This patient has paranoid ideation.

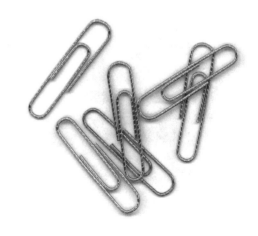

Decision Point E

Feature	Good prognosis	Bad prognosis
E1. Younger onset		+2
E2. Good premorbid interpersonal function	+2	
E3. Poor social supports		+2
E4. Short active psychotic phase	+2	
E5. Family history of schizophrenia		+2
E6. Family history of mood disorders	+2	
E7. Multiple relapses		+2
E8. Insidious onset		+2
E9. Prolonged active psychotic phase		+2
E10. Prominent positive symptoms	+2	

In general, a diagnosis of schizophrenia is not favorable. Only 10%–20% of schizophrenic patients were judged to have a favorable outcome 5–10 years after their first hospitalization. Interestingly, despite the development of novel antipsychotic medications and treatments and improvements in outpatient treatment, the overall prognosis of schizophrenia has changed little over the past century. It is estimated that more than 50% of schizophrenic individuals have worsening of symptoms or "downward drift" (as patients are less functional in society, their ability to care for themselves deteriorates as does their ability to earn income, resulting in a downward social and economic drift; this phenomenon is responsible for the mistaken impression that this illness is relegated to those of lower socioeconomic status), episodes of mood disorder, and, as stated above, a higher than average suicide rate. According to Kaplan and Sadock et al. 40%–60% of schizophrenics remain severely impaired throughout life. Positive symptoms, such as delusional thinking, often diminish gradually after the fifth decade of life leaving only the negative, residual symptoms.

Within the subtypes of schizophrenia, the paranoid subtype has the best overall prognosis and later age of onset. It is more common to see earlier, more insidious onset of symptoms in disorganized or undifferentiated subtypes which have much worse prognoses.

Your Total

Decision Point	Score	Ideal Score
A		5
B		10
C		8
D		9
E		20
Total		52

Key Clinical Points

1. Patients presenting with severe and acute agitation should be treated with medications as quickly as possible to prevent harm to themselves or others.
2. When considering the etiology of patients' acute psychosis, regardless of historic diagnosis, the differential is broad, including neurological, infectious, metabolic, oncological, and immunological processes, as well as alcohol and drug intoxication or withdrawal and vitamin deficiency.
3. Good premorbid interpersonal function, a short active psychotic phase, a family history of mood disorders and prominent positive symptoms, are indicators of a better prognosis for patients diagnosed with schizophrenia.

References

Alaghband-Rad J, McKenna K, Gordon CT, Albus KE, Hamburger SD, Rumsey JM, Frazier JA, Lenane MC, Rapoport JL: Childhood-onset schizophrenia: the severity of premorbid course. J Am Acad Child Adolesc Psychiatry 1995; 34:1273–1283

Allen MH, Currier GW, Carpenter D, Ross RW, Docherty JP (Expert Consensus Panel for Behavioral Emergencies 2005). The expert consensus guideline series: Treatment of behavioral emergencies 2005. J Psychiatr Pract 2005; 11(suppl 1):5–108; quiz 110–112

American Psychiatric Association. Diagnostic and Statistical Manual of Mental Disorders, 4th ed, text revision. Washington, DC, American Psychiatric Association, 2000

American Psychiatric Association, American Psychiatric Nurses Association, National Association of Psychiatric Health Systems: Learning From Each Other: Success Stories and Ideas for Reducing Restraint/Seclusion in Behavioral Health. Arlington, VA, American Psychiatric Association, 2003

Bartels SJ, Drake RE. Depressive symptoms in schizophrenia: comprehensive differential diagnosis. Compr Psychiatry 1988; 29:467–483

Caine ED. Clinical perspectives on atypical antipsychotics for treatment of agitation (review). J Clin Psychiatry 2006; 67(suppl. 10):22–31

Cannon M, Caspi A, Moffitt TE, Harrington H, Taylor A, Murray RM. Evidence for early-childhood, pan-developmental impairment specific to schizophreni-form disorder: results from a longitudinal birth cohort. Arch Gen Psychiatry 2002; 59:449–456

Collaborative Working Group on Clinical Trial Evaluations. Atypical antipsychotics for treatment of depression in schizophrenia and affective disorders. J Clin Psychiatry 1998; 59(suppl 12):41–45

Dubin WR. Rapid tranquilization: antipsychotics or benzodiazepine? J Clin Psychiatry 1988; 49(suppl):5–12

Erlenmeyer-Kimling L, Cornblatt B, Friedman D, Marcuse Y, Rutschmann J, Simmens S, Devi F: Neurological, electrophysiological and attentional deviations in children at risk of schizophrenia, in Schizophrenia as a Brain Disease. Edited by Henn FA, Nasrallah HA. New York, Oxford University Press, 1982, pp 61–98

Gottesman II, Shields J. Schizophrenia: The Epigenetic Puzzle. Cambridge, UK, Cambridge University Press, 1982

Hill S, Petit J. The violent patient. Emerg Med Clin North Am 2000; 18:301–305

Hughes DH, Kleespies PM. Treating aggression in the psychiatric emergency service. J Clin Psychiatry 2003; 64(suppl 4):10–15

Hyman SE. The suicidal patient, in Manual of Psychiatric Emergencies, 3rd ed. Edited by Hyman SE, Tesar GE. Boston, Little, Brown, 1994, p. 144

Koreen AR, Siris SG, Chakos M, Alvir J, Mayerhoff D, Lieberman J. Depression in first-episode schizophrenia. Am J Psychiatry 1993; 150:1643–1648

Marder SR. A review of agitation in mental illness: treatment guidelines and current therapies (review). J Clin Psychiatry 2006; 67(suppl 10):13–21

Plomin R, Reiss D, Hetherington EM, How GW. Nature and nurture: genetic contributions to measures of the family environment. Dev Psychol 1994; 30:32–43

Radomsky ED, Haas GL, Mann JJ, Sweeney JA. Suicidal behavior in patients with schizophrenia and other psychotic disorders. Am J Psychiatry 1999; 156:1590–1595

Robson KS (ed). Manual of Clinical Child and Adolescent Psychiatry, rev. ed. Washington, DC, American Psychiatric Press, Inc, 1994

Rund DA, Ewing JD, Mitzel K, Votolato N. The use of intramuscular benzodiazepines and antipsychotic agents in the treatment of acute agitation or violence in the emergency department (review). J Emerg Med 2006; 31:317–324

Sadock BJ, Sadock VA. Kaplan and Sadock's Comprehensive Textbook of Psychiatry, 8th ed. Philadelphia, Lippincott Williams & Wilkins, 2005

Salzman C, Green Al, Rodriguez-Villa F, Jaskiw Gl. Benzodiazepines combined with neuroleptics for management of severe disruptive behavior. Psycho-somatics 1986; 27:17–22

San L, Arranz B, Escobar R. Pharmacological management of acutely agitated schizo-phrenic patients (review). Curr Pharm Des 2005; 11:2471–2477

Sands JR, Harrow M. Depression during the longitudinal course of schizophrenia. Schizo-phr Bull 1999; 25:157–171

Simpson JC, Tsuang MT. Mortality among patients with schizophrenia. Schizophr Bull 1996; 22:485–499

Siris SG. Depression in schizophrenia: perspective in the era of "atypical" antipsychotic agents. Am J Psychiatry 2000; 157:1379–1389

Walker E, Lewis N, Loewy R, Palyo S. Motor dysfunction and risk for schizophrenia. Dev Psychopathol 1999; 11:509–523

Walker EF, Savoie T, Davis D. Neuromotor precursors of schizophrenia. Schizophr Bull 1994; 20:441–451

Watt N, Saiz C. Longitudinal studies of premorbid development of adult schizophrenics, in Schizophrenia: A Life-Course Developmental Perspec-tive. Edited by Walker E. San Diego, Academic Press, 1991, pp 158–185

Woods SW, Millar TJ, Davidson L, Hawkins KA, Sernyak MJ, McGlashan TH. Estimated yield of early detection of prodromal or first episode patients by screening first-degree relatives of schizophrenic patients. Schizophr Res 2001; 52:21–27

Yildiz A, Sachs GS, Turgay A. Pharmacological management of agitation in emergency settings. Emerg Med J 2003; 20:339–346

2

Bipolar Disorder

I'm Afraid He's Going to Quit His Job for No Reason

VIGNETTE PART I

"I realize now that I've got some major problems and I want to work with you so I can get better. Can I see you weekly?" The patient, Mr. J, shakes your hand with a firm grip, sits down, and immediately begins eating the hard candy from the bowl beside his chair as if he has not eaten all day. "I am still in a partial day program, but I want to wean myself slowly from that intensity by transitioning to weekly outpatient treatments. What do you think?"

You are an adult psychiatrist in independent practice, and this patient was referred to you by a colleague who runs an adult inpatient psychiatric service at the local hospital and who tells you that the patient is ready to move on to individual therapy. He feels that the patient no longer meets the criteria for his day program.

Mr. J is a 52-year-old recently divorced engineer, father of a son and a daughter, both in college. He was hospitalized for the first time after he was brought to an emergency room by ambulance, disheveled, in clothes he apparently had not changed in a week or more, angrily ranting that his wife was a "whore" and "the DEA is after me." According to the hospitalization notes you received with the patient's permission, his sister feared he was going to kill himself, after he made threats to do so, and she called for an ambulance. Three weeks before hospitalization, his son moved out of the house and in with his mother (the patient's ex-wife) because of fears his father was "losing control."

The patient spent 3 weeks as an inpatient, was started on quetiapine and quickly titrated to 300 mg TID, and fluoxetine titrated to 40 mg daily. After discharge he was admit-ted to the same hospital's day treatment program and spent the last 2 weeks there, attending groups and individual therapy for much of the day.

You begin by asking the patient to tell you about himself. "I am the lead engineer at a major construction firm here in town. I've been with this company for 24 years and I basically built it. It used to be a small operation and now we're handling contracts worth $20–50 million. That is all me. My staff grew from two assistants to a staff of about 25 people. I have one boss who is probably my best friend. I have two kids in school, but it was my wife that started this whole thing. My wife and my son's friend. Well, he's a friend of mine, too. But really, I need to reevaluate that whole relationship. I'm sure I'm in deep shit about it now, but I finally realized that there's nothing I can do." He looks at you, his eyebrows raised. Then he scans the corners of the ceiling without moving his head. "Is there? I mean, if they're going to come for me, then they're going to come for me. It is what it is. This is completely confidential, right?"

You tell him that what you talk about is completely confidential unless he makes specific threats for which you have a duty to warn. "Well, if they really want to know something from you I doubt you'd be able to stop them anyway. They're the government." You ask about the incident that led to his hospitalization. "There's no simple way to put this." With a sigh, he opens another piece of candy. "Let me see if I can sum it up for you: My wife cheated on me, and one of my colleagues—someone I trusted—really . . . well, you are a doctor . . . she gave me herpes and then lied about it. But I know it was her. And Spence, well he's the reason I'm likely going to jail. And I probably should not have let my daughter and her friends have beer over at the house."

His speech is rapid and he shifts frequently in his chair. "This medication, though, really helps. You should have seen me before. Since they started this stuff I've got my energy back big time." Beginning approximately 5–6 months earlier he became depressed. About 2 months later he came very close to quitting his job because he was certain they were monitoring his e-mail account and probably watching him with cameras placed strategically in the office, and he now knows he can trust only one other person there. "This is not my imagination," he insists. "You can tell when something is going on when people start behaving in a way that is very suspicious." He mentions an incident at a board meeting that took place in Florida at a golf resort, for a company with which he had landed a major contract just before the recent depressive episode. His main contact at that company is the woman he says gave him herpes. "I could see it in her eyes when I walked into the meeting. It was really obvious. From the moment I entered everyone stopped talking. I sat down next to her and she got up and moved to the other end of the table, supposedly to talk with one of her colleagues. But I know she was avoiding me. So I became angry." He laughs nervously. "I probably should not have let myself go like that. They all thought I was . . . well, I was actually . . . nuts."

Home from the meeting, he could not get out of bed "for days. I could not move. It was as if I was made out of lead. If I moved, it was to the sofa." Sometimes he watched the TV; sometimes he simply stared at the clock and watched it move hour after hour. "I had a talk show on the TV every day, but I cannot tell you any details beyond that. I remember thinking that this was a sign I was dying inside." He goes on: "I thought about all of the things I have done and several times I thought about killing myself." At his lowest point, he asked his sister to come over to his house and remove his pistol "just in case. But I think I really freaked out my son. He went back to live with my wife." Then he laughed to himself. "I called her 'my wife.' I seem to do that still. She's not. Not after what she did to me. That was the last straw." He continued to be depressed with suicidal ideation until "things just fell off the deep end," and he was taken to the hospital.

Today he is not suicidal. "I do think about it, but it is much less than I had been doing." Nor is he homicidal. He says he never heard any voices or saw any visual hallucinations, never thought the TV or radio was speaking to him, "but if you are asking me if I'm paranoid, I may be. But it is real. People really are watching me. I can prove it." He asks you to reiterate that your sessions are confidential, which you do. "I probably did some things I should not have, like keeping copies of certain e-mails and memos, copies of plans, and some

other things I will not mention. I stored them away. I also stored away other bits of evidence, especially the e-mails I wrote to my friend in California. He used to be a big druggie back when we were in college. I'm sure that is the connection the DEA is going to use to put me away."

Since taking the quetiapine, he is getting approximately 8–10 hours of sleep per night. At first he felt groggy from the medication, but now does not feel any morning "hangover." Right now he does not feel he can handle work, although he plans to return. But he thinks he might get fired in any event. His energy has improved, but he still has difficulty watching an entire TV program and has not read a book in months. His appetite is "tremendous," but he thinks that has something to do with the medication. "Do you think there is another medication I could try that will not give me such an appetite?" He does not recall ever going without sleep and tells you that he always talks this fast.

Your session ends, and he asks if he can return in 2 or 3 days instead of waiting a whole week.

DECISION POINT A

Given what you know about this patient from the limited history and first session and assuming you can fit him into your schedule as he requested, would you offer him an appointment in 2–3 days as requested?

A1. _____ Offer the additional appointment. But tell him you will only do this one time because he is also receiving psychiatric care at the partial hospitalization day program.

A2. _____ Offer the additional appointment. But tell him you only see patients with his type of illness once per week, so you will only do this one time. Your job is to provide medical management. Offer to refer him to a psychologist or social worker for psychotherapy.

A3. _____ Offer the additional appointment. Tell him you are happy to see him twice per week if he feels he needs the extra support.

A4. _____ Offer the additional appointment but only if either he can pay out of pocket or if his insurance will cover the cost of the additional visit.

A5. _____ Do not offer the additional appointment. Tell him that he is still in a partial hospitalization day program and you will not be able to offer him better services than he is already receiving.

A6. _____ Do not offer the additional appointment. Tell him that you are the doctor and you will decide whether he needs to see you more than once per week. If you feel he needs extra appointments, you will let him know.

DECISION POINT B

Given what you know about this patient, what is your differential diagnosis? Include rule-outs. (+2) points for correct answers, (−2) points for incorrect answers.

AXIS I:	
AXIS II:	

VIGNETTE PART II

Over the next 2 weeks the patient comes twice weekly for appointments. You hear more details about how the DEA is likely to arrest him for his connection to a friend from college he has not seen in more than 25 years who works as a neurologist and who may or may not be using drugs. "My daughter is having trouble at school, staying up all night and unable to work. She's like me in some ways," he tells you. There was a party he let his daughter have at his house with her girlfriends, all of whom were 18–19 years of age. He allowed them to have beer and feels guilty about that. There is a small collection of pornographic magazines "from years ago" that he recently put into a plastic box to store along with the e-mails and other items he brought home from his office. Spence, his son's friend, will soon be in trouble for getting caught outside a fraternity party smoking a marijuana joint, Mr. J suddenly explains, although Spence and his friends were only given warnings by the campus police.

You have trouble redirecting him. "I have so much to tell you," he responds. "I need to get this all out or you will not understand how deep this stuff is." His wife, for example, never cared about him. She had "the gall" to tell him about her affairs. "I do not know how many she had. She would go out of the house and say, 'Yes, I'm going out with another man.' I just could not take that anymore, so one night I had the locks changed as soon as she left. She went to stay with my sister." They divorced in the last 6 months. Then he admits they are not actually divorced but separated. "I bought her a house across the lake from me. She wants us to stay in close proximity because of the kids."

He tells you the surveillance at work is getting worse. "I went in, just to check things out. My boss said I can have this time off, but I wanted to see if anything had changed around

my desk." Suddenly smiling, he nods his head. "I could not get into my e-mail. I know they tampered with it. And everyone seems to know what happened to me, although I asked my boss not to say anything." He still attends the day program at the hospital, but they want him to reduce the amount of time he spends there and try to manage his problems with you.

"Actually, I'm starting to have trouble sleeping. I have so many thoughts spinning around my head. There have been too many hang-up calls, though," he insists. "I asked Spence to come with me to the place where I put all of the evidence, and there is one box missing. I know he took it. I think he's going to use it to frame me. I do not know. I'm going to have to do something. Confront him, I guess. But I cannot have him come around the house anymore. I'm not suicidal or homicidal, he recounts. I'm not even depressed, really." He tells you that Spence liked to use his piano.

He tells you he decreased the amount of quetiapine he takes to 600 mg because he's gaining weight and he's feeling "hung over" in the mornings.

DECISION POINT C

You are concerned about the level of paranoia, which seems to be escalating. What changes, if any, would you make to his medication regimen?

C1. _____ Increase dose of quetiapine to 1200 mg.

C2. _____ Maintain quetiapine at the current level and discontinue fluoxetine.

C3. _____ Increase quetiapine back to 900 mg, keep fluoxetine at the current level, and augment the quetiapine with risperidone, beginning at

1 mg qHS and titrating by 1 mg every 2–3 days until psychotic symptoms abate or a maximum of 6 mg.

C4. _____ Maintain quetiapine at the current level, discontinue fluoxetine, and augment the quetiapine with risperidone, beginning at 1 mg qHS and titrating by 1 mg every 2–3 days until psychotic symptoms abate or a maximum of 6 mg.

C5. _____ Maintain quetiapine at the current level, discontinue fluoxetine, augment the quetiapine with risperidone, beginning at 1 mg qHS and titrating by 1 mg every 2–3 days until psychotic symptoms abate or a maximum of 6 mg. Ask for permission to speak with his sister, ex-wife, and children.

C6. _____ Maintain medications as they are, but ask for permission to speak with his sister, ex-wife, and children before making any changes.

VIGNETTE PART III

You make the appropriate changes to his medication regimen, and his paranoia abates to what you estimate to be 20% of what it was. His affect seems calmer and his thoughts are more linear and goal-directed. The patient consents to allow you to speak with his sister, ex-wife, and children. His children are unavailable, but his sister and ex-wife arrive with the patient at his next visit. His sister is visibly upset, becoming tearful. She asks to see you alone first. "I'm so scared," she tells you. "I think what you are doing is working as long as he takes his medications. But I worry he'll stop taking them again and I do not want him to kill himself. I'm also afraid he's going to quit his job for no good reason. You have to understand, his boss loves him. Whatever he might have told you about that firm being so successful because of my brother is true. He has always been a workaholic. They probably take advantage of him for that, but he loves what he does. They're patient. They'll wait for him to be ready to return to work. But I do not understand what's happening to him. His wife never cheated on him. I do not know where that comes from. She does not want a divorce, either. That is why she lives across the lake. She loves him. Did he tell you that she makes him dinner every night still?"

She does not know if their parents had mental illness because they were both adopted. His daughter, however, recently started seeing a psychiatrist for bipolar disorder. You ask if she can recall the first time the patient may have had any mood symptoms. "He used to get depressed when we were kids. It would not last too long, but I remember times when he would go to his room and we could not get him out of there." Then her eyes light up. "I never told anyone about this. When J. was about 18 or 19, I remember going to a grocery store with him and he started saying, 'They're watching me. They're watching me.' I did not know if he was kidding or not. But he kept saying it to himself. I asked him about it and he denied the whole thing. Do you think that may have been something?"

The patient and his ex-wife enter the room. You gently ask the patient if it is true that he has dinner with his ex-wife every night. "Yeah," he replies. "She has been the one rock in my life throughout this whole ordeal." You ask him about college. "I've always been the sort of guy who has to get things done. You asked me if I ever went without sleep and I did not. I always got some sleep. But often that was just 2 or 3 hours if I had lots of work to do. I was president of the engineering fraternity, in the honor society, I had a few different girlfriends at the time, and I even started a small business venture with a friend of mine. I do not know how I did it." He says he never felt as though he had special powers or gifts, but "I was the guy people came to when they needed anything." He denied ever going into large amounts of debt because he managed to make a lot of money as a college student through his own business, but he did travel to different countries in Europe, Japan, Hawaii, and he owned a used Porsche. "I could think of several things at the same time and manage them somehow. When I was a kid I always had trouble focusing on any single thing. I always had a three to four things going at the same time." His sister nods.

DECISION POINT D

The medication change you made was to maintain the quetiapine at 600 mg, maintain the fluoxetine at 40 mg, and augment the quetiapine with risperidone 4 mg qHS. Given what you learned subsequently from the patient, his progress, and collateral information from his sister regarding his past history and present condition, what changes, if any, would you make to your primary diagnosis?

D1. _____ Brief psychotic disorder
D2. _____ Major depression, recurrent, severe with psychotic features
D3. _____ Bipolar I disorder, most recent episode manic, with psychotic features
D4. _____ Bipolar II disorder, most recent episode depressed, with psychotic features
D5. _____ Mood disorder with psychotic features

DECISION POINT E

Based upon your answer to Decision Point D, what changes, if any, would you make to his medication regimen?

E1. _____ Keep everything the same for now.
E2. _____ Slowly cross-taper the quetiapine with lithium or valproate, and maintain the fluoxetine at 40 mg and risperidone at 4 mg for now. Once the patient is off quetiapine, start to wean him from risperidone.
E3. _____ Discontinue the quetiapine and start either lithium or valproate. Maintain the risperidone at 4 mg and fluoxetine at 40 mg for now.
E4. _____ Discontinue the fluoxetine immediately, main-

tain the quetiapine at 600 mg and risperidone at 4 mg and start lithium or valproate. Once the patient is stable with either mood stabilizer, slowly wean him from quetiapine.

E5. _____ Slowly cross-taper the quetiapine with lithium or valproate, and discontinue the risperidone and fluoxetine.

DECISION POINT F

Most bipolar disorders begin with depressed episodes, subsequently making the distinction between bipolar or unipolar depressions difficult to diagnose. Which of the following differences in phenomenology between bipolar and unipolar depression are more common in bipolar disorder?

F1. _____ Atypical symptoms (increased sleep, increased appetite, rejection sensitivity, leaden paralysis, and mood reactivity without marked anhedonia)

F2. _____ Psychosis

F3. _____ Depressed mixed state (major depression with manic symptoms that are subthreshold for DSM-IV-TR definition, such as increased psychomotor activity, racing or crowded thoughts, and periods of decreased need for sleep)

F4. _____ Anxious/agitated depression (the presence of concurrent anxiety in the absence of manic symptoms)

DECISION POINT G

Which of the following differences in the course of illness are more suggestive of a bipolar depression rather than unipolar depression?

G1. _____ Early age at onset

G2. _____ Recurrence

G3. _____ Postpartum

G4. _____ Rapid cycling

G5. _____ Brief duration of depressive episodes

G6. _____ Baseline hyperthymic personality

ANSWERS: SCORING, RELATIVE WEIGHTS, AND COMMENTS

High positive scores (+3 and above) indicate a decision that would be effective, would be required for diagnosis, and without which management would be negligent. Lower positive scores (+2) indicate a decision that is important but not immediately necessary. The lowest positive score (+1) indicates a decision that is potentially useful for diagnosis and treatment. A neutral score (0) indicates a decision that is neither helpful nor harmful under the given circumstances. High negative scores (−5 to −3) indicate a decision that is inappropriate and potentially harmful or possibly life-threatening. Loser negative scores (−2 and above) indicate a decision that is nonproductive and potentially harmful.

DECISION POINT A

This question requires the reader to consider how willing he or she is to take on what may be a complicated case. It is true that as a psychiatrist you are responsible for the medical management of this patient and are not required to engage the patient in any psychotherapy. However, if you have the skill sets to offer even supportive psychotherapy, there is no need to spread this patient's care around to too many clinicians. It is true that he is already in a partial hospitalization day treatment program; however, your colleague, who runs the program, has referred the patient to you because he no longer meets the criteria to remain in that setting.

If you have the ability to offer biweekly sessions to this patient, there is no reason not to do so. However, if you feel that the reason the patient wishes to see you biweekly is a transference issue, you must confront your countertransference and determine the sort of relationship you feel is appropriate, necessary, or inappropriate and perhaps unnecessary. Do you wish to see this patient more frequently than once per week? You also might consider a weaning schedule, as he suggested, beginning biweekly and then tapering to once per month or more once the patient is stable.

Consider here the fact that the patient's symptoms are still somewhat unstable. There is a lot of history and collateral information missing to make an accurate diagnosis at this early stage in a patient with such a complex presentation.

A1. _____ −5 The patient was referred to you because he no longer meets the criteria for the partial day hospitalization program.

A2. _____ −3 You may not want to see the patient every week, and because of your own limitations, whether time or the ability to offer yet-to-be-determined therapy. However, you should not tell him how you treat his "kind of illness." This statement can be construed as pejorative, especially in a patient who presents in such a fragile state.

A3. _____ +4 Because there is no "right" answer, only 4 points are given here. This certainly is the most ambitious approach and will allow you to help the patient both with diagnosis and subsequent treatment in a more intensive and possibly rapid fashion, which is his desire.

A4. _____ 0 This answer is neither right nor wrong. It is a sad fact about our health care system, and more specifically, about mental health benefits.

A5. _____ −4 Again, he is being discharged from the former treatment. Being confrontational about his needs in this case will probably hurt your therapeutic alliance. However, setting limits is often helpful.

A6. _____ −5 This answer is needlessly paternalistic with an offensive, punitive tone.

DECISION POINT B

DIFFERENTIAL DIAGNOSIS

AXIS I:	(−5) Brief Psychotic Disorder (+3) Schizophrenia, Paranoid Type (+5) Schizophreniform Disorder (−5) Schizoaffective Disorder (−5) Delusional Disorder, grandiose type (−5) Delusional Disorder, jealous type (−5) Delusional Disorder, persecutory type (−5) Delusional Disorder, mixed type (+5) Major Depressive Disorder with psychotic features (+3) Bipolar I Disorder, most recent episode manic, severe with psychotic features (−5) Bipolar II Disorder, most recent episode hypomanic, severe with psychotic features
AXIS II:	(−5) Schizotypal Personality Disorder (−5) Narcissistic Personality Disorder

Brief Psychotic Disorder (−5). This patient's psychotic symptoms, including paranoia, possible delusions of grandeur, jealousy, persecution, began 2 months after the onset of depression and lasted approximately 4 months before his hospitalization. According to DSM-IV-TR, for brief psychotic disorder his symptoms, including the presence of one or more of the following—delusions, hallucinations, disorganized speech, grossly disorganized, or catatonic behavior—must have lasted between 1 day and 1 month with eventual return to premorbid functioning and not be better accounted for by another psychiatric disorder, medical condition, or substance effect.

Schizophrenia, Paranoid Type (+3). The patient elaborated at least 4 months' worth of delusions, including possible grandeur, jealousy, and persecution, has rapid speech, which he tells you is his baseline, seems to have some looseness of associations in his initial presentation despite treatment with quetiapine, and was brought to the emergency room grossly disorganized, "disheveled, in clothes he apparently had not changed in at least a week or more, and angrily ranting that his wife was a 'whore' and 'the DEA is after me'." To meet DSM-IV-TR criteria for criterion A symptoms, he requires two or more of delusions, hallucinations, disorganized speech, grossly disorganized or catatonic behavior, and negative symptoms. He certainly met the criteria of delusions and disorganization. His delusions, however, were not bizarre, nor did he have hallucinations of a voice keeping up a running commentary on the person's behavior or thoughts or two or more voices conversing with each other, of which only one is required to meet criterion A.

He did suffer from social/occupational dysfunction, worrying that both he and his activities (work, personal life, and e-mail:) were under surveillance and he would be caught at any time, meeting criterion B. More information would be required to determine if the "prodrome" of depression that occurred before the onset of psychotic symptoms would include only negative symptoms or two or more of the symptoms in criterion A in an attenuated form. Although this may seem unlikely, especially because this patient does not exhibit a reactive affect and his depression is described in terms more consistent with a classic, neurovegetative depression, this cannot yet be ruled out. Subsequently, it is not possible to say that the entire episode lasted at least 6 months, satisfying the duration requirement of criterion C.

Criterion D requires the ruling out of *schizoaffective disorder and mood disorder with psychotic* features. The patient describes his psychosis as having occurred 2 months after the onset of a major depressive episode, which continued concurrently. The duration of the major depression occurred during the entirety of the subsequent 4 months of worsening psychosis.

There is no evidence of substance abuse or medical illness that could explain his symptoms (criterion E), and although you would require more detailed history to ascertain whether he had a history of autistic disorder or other pervasive disorder, this seems unlikely given his success in both his career and social life (married with two grown children, many friends, and the ability to "land a major contract") before the onset of the current illness (criterion F).

The paranoid subtype requires that he have a preoccupation with one or more delusions or frequent auditory hallucinations and that none of the following is prominent: disorganized speech, disorganized or catatonic behavior, or flat or inappropriate affect. Until collateral information can be obtained, the delusions of grandeur and jealousy may not be psychotically derived, although his worries about the extent to which his life is being monitored and the imminence of his arrest by the DEA or other authority is a stronger argument for a delusion of persecution. Subsequently, you cannot yet make this distinction.

Schizophreniform Disorder (+5). Criterion A of schizophreniform disorder requires that criteria A, D, and E of schizophrenia be met, which is the case. Criterion B requires that the duration of the episode is at least 1 month but less than 6 months. The patient met the criteria for at least 4 months before treatment.

Schizoaffective Disorder (−5). See comment about schizophrenia criterion B above.

Delusional Disorder, Grandiose Type, Jealous Type, Persecutory Type, or Mixed Type (−5). Although the delusions of grandiosity and jealousy or persecution are not considered bizarre (criterion A), because criterion A for schizophrenia *was* met, that rules out delusional disorder. Additionally, for delusional disorder, his functioning must not be markedly impaired (criterion C), and the mood episodes must have been brief in duration relative to the totality of the delusional symptoms (criterion D), neither of which was the case. Criterion E states that the delusion must not have been better accounted for by the direct physiological effects of a substance or a general medical condition.

Major Depressive Disorder with Psychotic Features (+5). The patient meets both the criteria for psychosis, experiencing approximately 4 months of worsening symptoms, and by his account, a depressed mood, most of the day, nearly every day, with increasing anhedonia and isolation, hyper-somnia, psychomotor retardation, loss of energy, poor concentration, and recurrent suicidal ideation for approximately 6 months. His symptoms caused his inability to work or engage others socially. These symptoms were not due to substances or a medical condition and were not accounted for by bereavement. It is therefore appropriate to diagnose a major depressive episode.

Bipolar I Disorder, Most Recent Episode Manic, Severe with Psychotic Features (+3). The patient describes a major depressive episode as discussed above. For bipolar I disorder, in addition to the major depression, it is possible he experienced a distinct period of abnormally and persistently elevated, expansive, or irritable mood for at least 1 week, although he did not specifically state this. The other caveat to criterion A that is met is hospitalization, although the presenting complaint was related to suicidal ideation, gross disorganization, and psychotic symptoms. What confounds the presentation of bipolar depression is that it may be unipolar depression with psychotic features. More history is required to determine the type of depression; however, his presentation in your office is more suggestive of hypomania or mania.

His statements about how important he is to his company and how he built it from a very small business into a multimillion dollar enterprise ("that is all me") suggest an inflated self-esteem. He denied having periods of not needing sleep, but he did not describe the more accurate symptom of decreased *need* for sleep. He was hyperverbal in your office, taking over from the minute he arrived. His story seemed loose at times, suggesting a flight of ideas, although it was not pressured. He describes being easily distracted, and without further information about his marriage, it seems there were enough problems with infidelity (whether his wife actually cheated on him or not, he contracted herpes during an affair), suggesting some increase in goal-directed behaviors or excessive involvement in pleasurable activities that have a high potential for painful consequences.

The patient was started on fluoxetine, a selective serotonin reuptake inhibitor (SSRI), which may have caused him to "flip" into a manic state once treatment started. If his depression was a bipolar and not a unipolar depression, then the likelihood of his becoming manic with the addition of fluoxetine is high.

However, as recent studies suggest that bipolar or schizophrenic depressed patients have less insight into their illnesses than do unipolar depressed patients, it is imperative to obtain collateral information about possible manic or hypomanic episodes. These patients are subsequently, almost by definition, unable to give an accurate account of such episodes. As a result, unless you witness first-hand over time a manic or hypomanic episode, you cannot confidently diagnose bipolar disorder without collateral information, which, in this patient, you do not yet have.

Bipolar II Disorder, Most Recent Episode Hypomanic, Severe with Psychotic Features (−5). The patient describes his manic symptoms as lasting longer than the 4 days that distinguishes bipolar II from bipolar I disorders. However, by definition, bipolar II disorder cannot feature psychosis.

Note: To more confidently diagnose an axis II disorder, ideally a clinician should wait until he or she has known the patient for a while and preferably not while the patient concurrently has an axis I disorder.

Schizotypal Personality Disorder (−5). Although this patient has delusions of paranoia, they are not bizarre or odd, he did not describe any unusual perceptual experiences, he spoke rapidly, but not demonstrative of odd thinking or speech, and his affect and behavior were not odd, eccentric, or peculiar. He did become paranoid and suspicious of others, but he previously had good relationships with peers, was married, had children, and worked partly as a salesman. This excludes the social and interpersonal deficits required for schizotypal personality disorder.

Narcissistic Personality Disorder (−5). There is no evidence of a pervasive pattern of grandiosity, a need for admiration, or a lack of empathy. What is described by the patient thus far is a fairly well-balanced, fruitful life that fell apart because of either a mood disorder or a psychotic disorder. More evidence, especially from collateral sources who have known the patient for a long period of time is required to make such a diagnosis. One might suggest "strong narcissistic personality traits," although this would do a disservice to the patient and to those caring for him as it would create a damaging label. Without further evidence to the contrary, the patient's personality style in this case seems more a reaction to his underlying mood or psychotic disorder.

DECISION POINT C

C1. _____ −3 When the patient was receiving a higher dose of this medication, he did not tolerate it well and subsequently decreased his own dose.

C2. _____ +3 Removing the SSRI with a high level of antipsychotic coverage may be enough to eliminate the manic symptoms, although in this case you should be wary of the very long half-life of fluoxetine. In the outpatient setting, you should make medication changes one at a time to determine the effect of each change. However, given the manic symptoms you witness in your office, plus the symptoms suggestive of bipolar disorder, especially in the context of the new addition of an SSRI, you should consider discontinuing the SSRI because studies have demonstrated that antidepressants, especially SSRIs and tricyclic antidepressants, appear to cause acute manic episodes in approximately 20%–50% of patients with bipolar depression type I more than in patients with type II.

C3. _____ −3 If the intention is to cross-taper the patient to risperidone because you prefer this atypical antipsychotic drug over quetiapine, which coincides with the Clinical Antipsychotic Trials of Intervention Effectiveness (CATIE) study results for the treatment of schizophrenic psychosis, you would not increase the quetiapine. However, other considerations in choosing risperidone include significant weight gain and a higher risk of extrapyramidal side effects.

C4. _____ +1 Augmenting the quetiapine with risperidone has not been demonstrated by any study to be more effective than cross-tapering to a different agent, especially as quetiapine was not tried at its maximum dosing, given the patient's ability to tolerate it. However, patient response to medication is often idiosyncratic and despite a lack of evidence for augmentation, patients may respond positively to an augmentation strategy for a variety of reasons, some of which are the new constellation of receptor activity and a placebo effect. As stated in C3, the increased risk of significant side effects must be considered. Discontinuing fluoxetine may have a positive effect in reducing manic symptoms, but this is not guaranteed, either, especially because you have not made the clear diagnosis of bipolar disorder.

C5. _____ −2 See above. What is more effective about this answer than those above it is the determination to obtain the necessary collateral information required to make your diagnosis and thereby guide your treatment.

C6. _____ +3 It is very important to recruit the support of family members, especially as you are trying to stabilize his psychiatric condition. If you see the patient twice per week, and he maintains his current condition, he is not in any danger. This may be the safest route. However, the patient is not stable and does require some medication adjustment. The risk for suicide in a patient with bipolar disorder or schizophrenia is high enough to warrant extreme caution.

DECISION POINT D

D1. _____ −5 See answers for Decision Point B.

D2. _____ −5 See answers for Decision Point B.

D3. _____ +5 With the collateral information, this patient clearly has a long history of manic symptoms and depressions dating back to his teen years. Because he was adopted, you cannot determine whether his relatives have mental illness; but his daughter has bipolar disorder. The likelihood of his also having bipolar disorder with one first-degree relative (his daughter) diagnosed with bipolar disorder is approximately 25%. He is one of those fortunate individuals who was long able to channel his diminished need for sleep, grandiosity, and other manic symptoms into a highly productive career. On the other hand, his hypomania became mania and eventually, because of lack of treatment, evolved into psychosis. His personal and professional life, as a result, suffered greatly. He may have concurrent cluster B personality traits such as narcissism, but this is more a personality style secondary to a primary mood disorder. In our society, persons who are overachievers, earn a lot of money, help others further their own careers or interests, and are ebullient, charismatic, and confident are held in high esteem. These traits are not necessarily pathological; however, when pathological symptoms are overlooked, these individuals can potentially cause great harm to themselves and others. We cannot lose sight of the 15%–20% suicide rate for individuals with untreated bipolar disorder.

D4. _____ −5 See answers for Decision Point B.

D5. _____ −5 See answers for Decision Point B.

DECISION POINT E

E1. _____ −5 The patient is clearly not stable with this drug regimen. Additionally, the quetiapine is not tolerated by the patient, so it should be discontinued if the dose cannot be maximized. Because the patient has bipolar disorder, treatment with a mood stabilizer should be started. The antidepressant should be discontinued immediately as this drug is most likely worsening his mood stability, causing anything from a mixed state to mania.

E2. _____ −4 Starting a mood stabilizer is the correct direction for this patient once he is stabilized.

However, maintaining the combination of quetiapine, which is intolerable to the patient, and fluoxetine, which is probably destabilizing his mood, is not recommended. If he is tolerating the lower dose of quetiapine, the combination with risperidone may be appropriate until the mood stabilizer is therapeutic. A better strategy would be to start the mood stabilizer and then slowly wean the patient from the atypical antipsychotic drug after the patient has been stable for at least a month.

E3. _____ −3 The fluoxetine should be discontinued. Discontinuing the quetiapine and starting lithium or valproate could work if the risperidone at 4 mg is able to stabilize the patient. This dose might need to be increased to 6 mg if the quetiapine is discontinued.

E4. _____ +4 Because this patient's medication regimen was already complicated, there is no perfect strategy. There are, however, some underlying principals about the treatment of bipolar disorder that are addressed by this combination. This patient needs a mood stabilizer. He should be maintained on an atypical antipsychotic drug until this is therapeutic. The atypical antipsychotic will help in the short run. An antidepressant should not be part of the regimen unless the patient has intolerably severe depression. In that case, one would probably choose bupropion because it has only a 15%–20% chance of "flipping" a patient into a mixed or manic state compared with other SSRIs that have a 30%–40% likelihood. Additionally, there are some findings in the current literature suggesting that the use of antidepressants in patients with bipolar disorder can cause them to develop a permanent rapid cycling mood disorder. The literature in this area is sparse, however, as randomized controlled studies examining this phenomenon have not yet been done.

E5. _____ +2 As long as the cross-taper is very slow and the patient tolerates this exchange of mood stabilizer for atypical antipsychotic, this is a possible solution. It would be safer, especially in the outpatient setting, to start the mood stabilizer with the atypical antipsychotic for support and then slowly taper the atypical antipsychotic.

DECISION POINT F

For the past 15–20 years, the literature has supported these symptoms as being more likely the phenomenology of a bipolar disorder. This suggests that diagnosing a bipolar mood disorder is easier than one might think, and given what is known about the difference in pharmacology, it is a very important distinction to make.

F1. _____ +2 Correct
F2. _____ +2 Correct
F3. _____ +2 Correct
F4. _____ +2 Correct

DECISION POINT G

As in Decision Point F, the literature supports these symptoms as being suggestive of a bipolar depressive course rather than a unipolar depressive course. It is important to make this distinction, especially in children and adolescents, because of the potential and significant dangers of giving antidepressants to children with bipolar disorder, which may "flip" them into mixed or manic states, and the suggestion that rapid cycling may be permanent.

G1. _____ +2 Correct
G2. _____ +2 Correct
G3. _____ +2 Correct
G4. _____ +2 Correct
G5. _____ +2 Correct
G6. _____ +2 Correct

YOUR TOTAL		
Decision Point	Your Score	Ideal Best Score
A		4
B		13
C		7
D		5
E		6
F		8
G		12
Total		55

Note: *The treatment options discussed above are based on a situation in which the patient is able to afford ideal medications, is not bothered by blood testing to monitor organ function, and will be reasonably compliant. He did decrease his quetiapine dose because of difficulty tolerating the medication; however, he did not discontinue it.*

In the real world, practitioners are faced with treatment decisions that often require consideration of the patient's socioeconomic status, compliance, and accessibility to health care, especially for ongoing monitoring of symptoms and blood testing. For example, when treating the patient with limited means or inadequate access to health care, one might be faced with a limited choice of medications; lithium carbonate might not be available. Instead, drug choices would be limited to divalproex, lamotrigine, or atypical neuroleptic drugs as primary agents, or they may be limited to the cheapest generic medications. A patient may refuse blood testing or not be reliable to have it done, necessitating the use of depot formulations of typical or atypical neuroleptics to give them as much relief of symptoms as possible.

KEY CLINICAL POINTS

1. Primary mood disorder with psychotic features is the likely diagnosis for a patient whose psychotic symptoms occur only in the presence of prominent mood symptoms.

2. Self-awareness and knowledge of one's own limits are key elements of professionalism. Once a doctor patient relationship is established, a physician may not ethically abandon the patient. If not able to provide the necessary care, the psychiatrist must assist in finding the proper resources for the patient.

3. Bipolar disorder can begin with a depressed episode and can be confused with unipolar depression; treatment with an antidepressant carries a significant likelihood that the patient may develop a mixed state. The physician must weigh the pros and cons of any medication before prescribing.

REFERENCES

Aksikal HS, Maser JD, Zeller PJ, Endicott J, Coryell W, Keller M, Warshaw M, Clayton P, Goodwin F: Switching from 'unipolar' to bipolar II: an 11-year prospective study of clinical and temperamental predictors in 559 patients. Arch Gen Psychiatry 1995; 52:114–123

Cassano GB, Akiskal HS, Savino M, Musetti L, Perugi G: Proposed subtypes of bipolar II and related disorders: with hypomanic episodes (or cyclothymia) and with hyperthymic temperament. J Affect Disord 1992; 26:127–140

Chiaroni P, Hantouche EG, Gouvernet J, Azorin JM, Akiskal HS: Hyperthymic and depressive temperaments study in controls, as a function of their familial loading for mood disorders. Encephale 2004; 30:509–515

El-Mallakh RS, Ghaemi SN: Bipolar Depression, a Comprehensive Guide. Washington, DC, American Psychiatric Association Publishing, 2006

Freeman MP, Keck PE Jr, McElroy SL: Postpartum depression with bipolar disorder. Am J Psychiatry 2001; 158:52

Geller B, Zimerman B, Williams M, Bolhofner K, Craney JL: Bipolar disorder at prospective follow-up of adults who had prepubertal major depressive disorder. Am J Psychiatry 2001; 158:125–127

Ghaemi SN, Hsu DJ, Ko JY, Baldassano CF, Kontos NJ, Goodwin FK: Bipolar spectrum disorder: a pilot study. Psychopathology 2004; 37:222–226

Ghaemi SN, Stoll AL, Pope HG: Lack of insight in bipolar disorder: the acute manic episode. J Nerv Ment Dis 1995; 183:464–467

Ghaemi SN, Boiman EE, Goodwin FK: Diagnosing bipolar disorder and the effect of antidepressants: a naturalistic study. J Clin Psychiatry 2000; 61:804–808

Ghaemi SN, Boiman EE, Goodwin FK: Diagnosing bipolar disorder and the effect of antidepressants: a naturalistic study. J Clin Psychiatry 2001; 62:565–569

Ghaemi SN, Rosenquist KJ, Ko JY, Baldassano CF, Kontos NJ, Baldessarini RJ: Antidepressant treatment in bipolar versus unipolar depression. Am J Psychiatry 2004; 161:163–165

Goldberg JF, Harrow M, Whiteside JE: Risk for bipolar illness in patients initially hospitalized for unipolar depression. Am J Psychiatry 2001; 158:1265–1270

Goodwin F, Jamison K: Manic Depressive Illness. New York, Oxford University Press, 1990

Henry C, Sorbara F, Lacoste J, Gindre C, Leboyer M: Antidepressant-induced mania in bipolar patients: identification of risk factors. J Clin Psychiatry 2001; 62:249–255

Judd LL, Akiskal HS, Maser JD, Zeller PJ, Endicott J, Coryell W, Paulus MP, Kunovac JL, Leon AC, Mueller TI, Rice JA: A prospective 12-year study of subsyndromal and syndromal depressive symptoms in unipolar major depressive disorders. Arch Gen Psychiatry 1998; 55:694–700

Keitner GI, Solomon DA, Ryan CE, Miller IW, Mallinger A, Kupfer DJ, Frank E: Prodromal and residual symptoms in bipolar I disorder. Compr Psychiatry 1996; 37:362–367

Kessing LV, Andersen PK, Mortensen PB: Recurrence in affective disorder, I: case register study. Br. J. Psychiatry 1998; 172:23–28

Mitchell P, Parker G, Jamieson K, Wilhelm K, Hickie I, Brodaty H, Boyce P, Hadzi-Palovic D, Roy K: Are there any differences between bipolar and unipolar melancholia? J Affect Disord 1992; 25:97–105

Mitchell PB, Wilhelm K, Parker G, Austin MP, Rutgers P, Malhi GS: The clinical features of bipolar depression: a comparison with matched major depressive disorder patients. J. Clin Psychiatry 2001; 62:212–216

Perlis RH, Smoller JW, Fava M, Rosenbaum JF, Nierenberg AA, Sachs GS: The prevalence and clinical correlates of anger attacks during depressive episodes in bipolar disorder. J Affect Disord 2004; 79:291–295

3

Major Depressive Disorder

My Life Doesn't Add Up

VIGNETTE PART 1

You are in private practice in adult psychiatry. You receive a phone call from Mr. D, who says he was referred to you by a colleague and asks if you are taking new patients. You ask him what he is hoping for, and he responds that he is "extremely depressed," that he just fired his previous psychiatrist because he "said some things that really bothered me" and "tried to force medications on me when he knows I've been able to manage my depressions with just therapy." You ask if this doctor also managed his psychotherapy. He says yes, they worked together for about 2 years, but Mr. D stopped meeting with him more than a year ago. You suggest that he make an appointment to come in and meet with you. His voice becomes angry. "I'm depressed," he says. "I'm not able to do my work. I can't think. I can't concentrate. I've been a mathematics professor for 22 years and for the first time I can't tell if I'm making any sense to my students. I don't think I can get myself to class today." You hear him crying. "I can't bear the idea of not doing my best and you want me to make an appointment?"

DECISION POINT A

Given this presentation, what is your next step? (Select the best answer. Points are taken away for incorrect answers.)

A1. _____ Tell Mr. D you would like to help him, but his anger will not allow you to do your evaluation efficiently.

A2. _____ Tell Mr. D you would like to help him, but you need more information. The only way to accomplish this is to meet with him in person to perform a thorough evaluation. Right now you do not have any available time, but you will gladly see him early next week.

A3. _____ Tell Mr. D you would like to help him, but you need more information. You are too busy to see him this week but you can refer him to a colleague who may have time in the next few days.

A4. _____ Ask Mr. D if he is thinking about hurting himself, or perhaps killing himself. If he answers in the affirmative, refer him to the psychiatric emergency room.

A5. _____ Ask Mr. D if he feels as though he needs to be seen immediately, and if so, refer him to the psychiatric emergency room.

A6. _____ Tell Mr. D that he still has a treatment relationship with his former psychiatrist and that he should contact him for a follow-up appointment.

VIGNETTE PART 2

Mr. D goes to the psychiatric emergency room. You are now the attending psychiatrist on duty and meet Mr. D for the first time. On evaluation you learn that he is 55 years old and has been feeling "depressed" for at least 3 years. He was elected president of his local teachers union about a year ago but had to quit the position 1 month ago because of "stress" and because he felt he was "not able to do the job the way it should be done." He is unable to sleep through the night; he has trouble initiating sleep and has middle insomnia. When he wakes up at night, which he does several times, he takes about a half-hour, sometimes more, to fall back asleep. Sometimes he stays up and tries to read or watch television, but, he says, "I can't follow anything. I can't stop my mind from running." His appetite is poor and he has lost 15 pounds unintentionally in the past month. His energy is low, and he feels as though he is "mired in muck." He is especially anxious about teaching. For the past 8 years he has consistently won the Teacher of the Year award at his college. Teaching mathematics is "automatic" at this point for him, but he feels as though he is not doing his best. Before he enters the classroom, he first has to convince himself that he can get through the lecture, but he still feels as though he is not making sense. He admits that it is possible that he may be doing a better job than he thinks, but he cannot help feeling as though he is letting his students down. He wonders if he should take time off.

He reports that he has suffered two previous bouts of major depression, 10 years ago after he and his wife separated, and 4 years ago after a job promotion. He overcame both episodes with psychotherapy alone. He and his wife are opposed to taking medications of any sort, including acetaminophen. "I don't know what you are going to propose to me, but I want you to know that I'm very skeptical of medications, especially fluoxetine." He tells you that his general practitioner gave him a prescription for fluoxetine 10 mg daily, but he did not fill it for fear that it would make him want to kill himself. He has been reading articles lately on the dangers of antidepressants, and he does not trust the drug companies, the government, or psychiatrists to level with him about the drugs' true risks.

He explains that his current depression reminds him of his previous two episodes of major depression, but now with more hopelessness and with suicidal ideation. "I know I don't want to do something stupid," he says, "but I can't get the thought out of my head." He admits to thinking about cutting his wrists and lying in a bathtub, shooting himself (he does not own a gun), and lying on railroad tracks. When he thinks about killing himself he feels "an adrenaline rush" because, he says, "I might go through with it, but it would devastate my family." He has been married for 25 years, and his wife has accompanied him to the psychiatric emergency room today. They have a son, 18, and a daughter, 22. You perform a Mini-Mental State Examination, and he scores 29/30, requiring prompting for recall.

DECISION POINT B

Given what you have learned so far, what would you most likely do next? (Select all that apply. Points are taken away for incorrect answers.)

B1. _____ Ask Mr. D where he heard about fluoxetine. What does he know about it? Then explain that it is a safe medication and that you'll give him some samples.

B2. _____ Tell him that you understand he is going through a great deal of stress right now with the teaching, the extra job he quit, and his worries about performance. Ask if there are any other issues that may be bothering him right now. Then tell him he has a more severe depressive disorder and this time he would respond best to medication and psychotherapy.

B3. _____ Ask specifically about his social supports. Whom would he call in an emergency?

B4. _____ Ask him about alcohol and drug consumption.

B5. _____ Explore the issue of ECT. Tell him this is probably his best bet if he wants a more effective, cheaper treatment than a lifetime on antidepressant medications.

B6. _____ Acknowledge that he felt some relief after psychotherapy with his previous bouts of major depression, but tell him you could have predicted he would be back for more intensive help, since psychotherapy is not a long-term solution to depression. Remind him that 15%–20% of cases of untreated depression end in suicide.

B7. _____ If the patient acknowledges that this bout is indeed different—especially more severe than before—or if he feels "helpless," gently suggest the availability of medications that are very effective against major depression.

B8. _____ Mention that sometimes you prescribe a benzodiazepine, one of the longer-acting ones, that can help him with his anxiety and that might make the weeks until the antidepressant kicks in more tolerable.

VIGNETTE PART 3

After long discussions, the patient and his wife agree that the severity of the current depression warrants a trial of pharmacological treatment. You discharge him with clonazepam 0.5 mg, which he should take twice daily, and 1 mg at bedtime as needed, and you tell him to fill the prescription for fluoxetine written by his primary care physician. Mr. D agrees to return in 1 week for a bridging appointment.

As agreed, Mr. D returns 1 week later. He tells you that he feels a little relief from the clonazepam but has been cutting your prescribed doses in half, as they were too sedating for him. He still feels depressed, hopeless, and worthless and still feels as though he is just going "through the motions" when he teaches and as though he is somehow letting his family down. His thoughts of suicide got worse for a few days at the beginning of the week, and he had some mild stomach ache, but his overall feeling has improved by now. He wonders if this fluoxetine is really going to work. He is also anxious to get started with a therapist, but it will be another 4 weeks before he can be seen by a therapist. He will have an appointment with his new psychiatrist in another 10 days.

DECISION POINT C

Given the above information, what would you do next? (Select all that apply. Points are taken away for incorrect answers.)

C1. _____ Tell him you are not going to give him any more clonazepam, because you do not want him to become addicted to it. He will need his regular psychiatrist to give him more than a week's worth.

C2. _____ Ask him if he has any other symptoms or side effects from the fluoxetine, and if not, suggest going up to fluoxetine 20 mg/day for now and make a bridging appointment for 1 week from today to meet with him one more time before his appointment with his new psychiatrist.

C3. _____ Tell him to finish out the prescription of clonazepam as you directed and say that you wouldn't give him too much on purpose.

C4. _____ Tell him to take as little clonazepam as he likes. He won't be hurt by taking smaller amounts. If he wants to take larger amounts, he should check with you first.

C5. _____ Agree with him that fluoxetine may not be working for him and tell him that there are many other antidepressants on the market. Provide him with literature on escitalopram and venlafaxine so he can make an informed decision.

C6. _____ Tell him to take some time off from work, as he probably will not be functioning at 100% until he makes a more complete recovery from his depression.

DECISION POINT D

The patient's therapist has many psychotherapeutic modalities from which to choose that may be useful in the treatment of major depressive disorder. The techniques and theories are individually defined for various purposes, including research and discussion. In practice, clinicians typically use a combination of techniques, depending on the patient's individual situation and coping capacities. Choose which psychotherapy modality is most closely identified with the following concepts. Each concept may have one or more answers.

	Psychodynamic Psychotherapy	Cognitive Behavior Psychotherapy	Dialectical Behavioral Therapy	Interpersonal Therapy	Supportive Psychotherapy
1. Turning anger back on the self					
2. All-or-nothing thinking					
3. Schedule of daily activities and pleasure					
4. Communication analysis					
5. Problem solving					
6. Absolutist, dichotomous thinking					
7. Exploring the psychological meaning of symptom formation					
8. Encouragement of affect					
9. Teaching of core mindfulness and emotion regulation skills					
10. Therapist as temporary substitute/auxiliary ego					

DECISION POINT E

Which of the following drugs are required to carry a black box warning urging families and physicians to monitor patients for "clinical worsening, suicidality, or unusual changes in behavior"?

A. _____ Clomipramine
B. _____ Trazodone
C. _____ Venlafaxine
D. _____ Amitriptyline
E. _____ Paroxetine
F. _____ Fluoxetine
G. _____ Bupropion
H. _____ Sertraline

ANSWERS: SCORING, RELATIVE WEIGHTS, AND COMMENTS

High positive scores (+3 and above) indicate a decision that would be effective, would be required for diagnosis, and without which management would be negligent. Lower positive scores (+2) indicate a decision that is important but not immediately necessary. The lowest positive score (+1) indicates a decision that is potentially useful for diagnosis and treatment. A neutral score (0) indicates a decision that is neither clearly helpful nor harmful under the given circumstances. High negative scores (−3 and above) indicate a decision that is inappropriate and potentially harmful or life-threatening. Lower negative scores (−2) indicate a decision that is nonproductive and potentially harmful. The lowest negative score (−1) indicates a decision that is not harmful but is nonproductive, time-consuming, and not cost-effective.

DECISION POINT A

A1. _____ −5 The patient is clearly angry and frustrated by his depression and his inability to work as he had done previously. Try to support his coming to you for help rather than adopting a paternalistic or defensive stance.

A2. _____ −2 This response acknowledges the patient's need for an appointment and his desire for help but not his frustration or his clearly fragile state.

A3. _____ +2 As in answer A2, this response acknowledges the patient's need for an appointment, and it also includes an attempt to facilitate an urgent appointment. However, since the patient is so emotionally labile, you should first explore whether he is in danger of hurting himself or others.

A4. _____ +5 This is a totally appropriate next step given the patient's frustration, his emotional lability, and his own acknowledgment that his mood and intentions are unpredictable.

A5. _____ +3 A similar response to A4 without closed questions that define his safety level.

A6. _____ −5 This is clearly not what Mr. D wants, and by brushing him off in this way you may harm the chances of other psychiatrists' forming a therapeutic alliance with him. You could later explore what went wrong in his previous treatment relationship, once the safety issues were properly managed.

DECISION POINT B

B1. _____ +1 You address one of his major concerns, but in your explanation of the safety of fluoxetine you may come across as forcing medications on the patient, which is precisely what drove him away from his previous psychiatrist.

B2. _____ +3 This answer contains a good reflection of the patient's key stressors and current mental state, which helps establish and strengthen the therapeutic alliance. Before announcing that "the other doctor was right," you should explore how nonpharmacological treatments

were effective for the patient and how previous episodes differ from the current presentation.

B3. _____ +5 Always a good question. If the patient is alone and does not have good social supports, his prognosis is much worse. His wife accompanied him, but it is never safe to assume a supportive marriage, especially given the history of a separation.

B4. _____ +5 Always ask. Both illnesses need treatment, as one certainly affects the other.

B5. _____ −5 ECT is known to have a higher rate of response in major depression than any other antidepressant treatment, especially in cases of moderate to severe depression that have not responded to pharmacological intervention. Approximately 50% of pharmacologically resistant depression will respond to ECT. The current method of applying this treatment is safe and effective. For this patient, because pharmacotherapy has not yet been tried and because the patient is still able to function, albeit with difficulty, ECT is not yet indicated—and even less so given his resistance to pharmacotherapy, which is somatically less invasive.

B6. _____ −5 It is true that 15%–20% of untreated depression ends in suicide, but the patient was being treated with psychotherapy, so this statistic does not apply. Additionally, telling him you could have predicted that he would require more treatment is inappropriate and untrue, and it could hurt your therapeutic alliance. The patient already said he was put off by his previous physician's being paternalistic.

B7. _____ +5 Good approach to the patient, acknowledging his current severe and perhaps very different presentation than in previous depressions as a means of "gently" broaching the subject of medications. The next step would be a brief psychopharmacology education, since this is an intellectually motivated individual.

B8. _____ +5 Again, this is appropriate once the patient is convinced that he should abandon the belief that he can overcome his depression without medications.

DECISION POINT C

C1. _____ −2 Since your disposition for this patient from the psychiatric emergency department included a bridging appointment to provide ongoing treatment and evaluation until he was able to make an appointment with a psychiatrist, you must be sure to refill his prescriptions as needed until another psychiatrist can take over the case. In this instance, you should find out how much clonazepam the patient has left and, if necessary, provide enough additional medication for another week. He is unlikely to become addicted to clonazepam with regular use during the first 2 weeks. Explain the potential for addiction, what the side effects of withdrawal are, and how withdrawal is treated.

C2. _____ +2 This is a reasonable option with the caveat that his clonazepam prescription must also be covered as mentioned in C1.

C3. _____ −2 If the clonazepam is helping him at the smaller dose, he should be encouraged to continue. He will not develop an addiction in such a short period given clonazepam's long half-life and the small dose. However, insisting that a patient "trust you" because "you are his doctor" is paternalistic. While some patients respond well to this approach, this patient already stated that he does not like it when a physician pressures him to take medication, so this should be avoided. You should react to the patient's questions as one who is allied with him such that you are working together in treatment.

C4. _____ +3 Discuss the pros and cons of smaller versus larger doses of clonazepam. Find out precisely what symptoms he is experiencing, and make specific suggestions about how to adjust the dose so that he has a firm understanding of how to proceed. Educating him will help him make his own decisions and subsequently feel empowered in his own treatment. He made it clear to you that he prefers not to take medications if possible. In this case he is likely to feel more confident about pharmacotherapy if he understands the concrete evidence you provide, and he will probably be comforted by your obvious understanding of his concerns.

C5. _____ −3 An adequate trial of an antidepressant, if there are no intolerable side effects, is 6 to 12 months. The onset of symptom relief will likely take 2 to 4 weeks in most individuals. Once you select an agent, you should stick with it unless the patient cannot tolerate it or it is clearly not effective.

C6. _____ 0 This should be a subject of discussion rather than a recommendation. The patient has said that he is having difficulty at work and that he has wondered about taking time off, but he does not convey the impression that he wishes to take time off. He mentioned that he is getting some relief from the clonazepam while the fluoxetine is just beginning to take effect.

DECISION POINT D

	Psychodynamic Psychotherapy	Cognitive Behavior Psychotherapy	Dialectical Behavioral Therapy	Interpersonal Therapy	Supportive Psychotherapy
1. Turning anger back on the self	+2				
2. All-or-nothing thinking		+2			
3. Schedule of daily activities and pleasure		+2			
4. Communication analysis				+2	
5. Problem solving		+2			+2
6. Absolutist, dichotomous thinking		+2			
7. Exploring the psychological meaning of symptom formation	+2				
8. Encouragement of affect				+2	+2
9. Teaching of core mindfulness and emotion regulation skills			+2		
10. Therapist as temporary substitute/auxiliary ego					+2

DECISION POINT E

As of October 15, 2004, all antidepressants prescribed in the United States are required by the Food and Drug Administration to carry the warning. The labeling also states that "although a causal link between the emergence of such symptoms and either the worsening of depression and/or the emergence of suicidal impulses has not been established, there is concern that such symptoms may represent precursors to emerging suicidality." (2 points for each correct answer.)

YOUR TOTAL

Decision Point	Your Score	Ideal Best Score
A		10
B		24
C		5
D		24
E		16
Total		79

KEY CLINICAL POINTS

1. Assessment of depressed patients always includes a thorough assessment of suicide risk.
2. A variety of psychotherapies demonstrate effectiveness in treating depression. Being flexible with one's technique will allow treatment of a greater range of patients.
3. A clear discussion of risks and benefits of medication prior to initiating a trial will enhance communication and compliance.

REFERENCES

American Psychiatric Association. Practice guideline for the treatment of patients with major depressive disorder, third edition. Am J Psychiatry 167 (Oct Suppl):1–118; 2010. Also available at http://psychiatryonline.com/pracGuide/pracGuideHome.aspx

American Psychiatric Association: Diagnostic and Statistical Manual of Mental Disorders, Fourth Edition, Text Revision. Washington DC, American Psychiatric Association, 2000

Sadock BJ, Sadock VA: Synopsis of Psychiatry, 10th ed. Philadelphia, Lippincott Williams & Wilkins, 2007

Shea SC: The Practical Art of Suicide Assessment. New York, Wiley, 2002

U.S. Food and Drug Administration (FDA) Website: Antidepressant Use in Children, Adolescents, and Adults: http://www.fda.gov/drugs/drugsafety/informationby-drugclass/ucm096273.htm

World Health Organization: World Health Report 2001: Mental Health: New Understanding, New Hope. Geneva, World Health Organization, 2001

4

Major Depressive Disorder and Suicide

I'm So Sick of This

VIGNETTE PART I

You are a psychiatrist in independent practice with a reputation for taking on challenging cases. You take on a case of a young woman, 28, single, with a past psychiatric history significant for borderline personality disorder, major depressive disorder, and panic disorder without agoraphobia. She has no previous psychiatric hospitalizations, but has been receiving outpatient psychotherapy and pharmacotherapy for the past 3 years. She is referred to you because her depressed mood has been treatment resistant. She calls and leaves a voice mail message on the Friday evening before her first appointment stating that she is "too depressed" to make it on Monday. She leaves a second message later that evening stating that she is feeling better and will make the appointment, apologizing profusely for her first message.

DECISION POINT A

Given what you have learned about this patient so far, is a decision to call the patient at home on a Friday evening at 9 p.m. appropriate? Points awarded for correct and incorrect answers are scaled from best (+5) to unhelpful but not harmful (0) to dangerous (−5).

A1. _____ No. Given the patient's prior psychiatric history of borderline personality disorder, you should consider the likelihood that she does not appreciate personal or professional borders. Calling her only rewards this inappropriate behavior.

A2. _____ No. The patient made it clear by her second message that she will make her appointment on Monday. You have not established a doctor-patient relationship at this point so you are not under any obligation to call her, especially at 9 p.m. on a Friday night.

A3. _____ No. The patient has a history of major depressive disorder and left a message that she is "too

depressed" to make an appointment 3 days hence. Then she called back to make it clear she felt better and would make her appointment on Monday. You have not established a doctor-patient relationship at this point so you are not under any obligation to call her. You do not know this patient except for the brief history that included borderline personality disorder. Calling her would reward her manipulative behavior.

A4. _____ Yes. The patient has a history of major depressive disorder and left a message that she is "too depressed" to make an appointment 3 days hence. Then she called back to make it clear she felt better and would make her appointment on Monday. Given that you do not know this patient and she expressed what may be understood as mood lability by her two messages, it would be prudent to check whether she is suicidal.

A5. _____ Yes. Although there is no evidence to support using the telephone with patients who are borderline for "coaching" in between visits, there is also no evidence that it is not appropriate or helpful. You do not know this patient except for her prior diagnoses and her two conflicting telephone messages that suggest mood instability. It would be appropriate to briefly establish a professional connection and check for suicidality.

VIGNETTE PART 2

You call her around 9 p.m. that same night to ask how she is feeling. You notice immediately that she is speaking slowly with a very soft voice.

"It's gone," she tells you. "I took a shower and listened to some music. I'm okay." You inquire further what she meant by "it's gone." She tells you that she was feeling helpless, hopeless, and started thinking about dying. "I know you don't know me yet, but I have been going through this . . . " Her words trail off; she begins to sob. You wait, and after a moment she says, "I'm so sorry. I'm really okay." You ask if she is thinking about harming herself or killing herself to which she calmly responds, "No. I'm solid. I haven't been to the hospital for this so far and I plan to keep it that way." She has the phone number for the local psychiatric emergency room and has called it numerous times to talk with a clinician when she starts to feel unsafe and this "always" helps her feel better. There are family members at home with her and she tells you she will not be alone. She tells you that when she feels this depressed she relieves the symptoms by taking a shower, listening to music, sitting in her backyard with a book, or writing in her journal. She also kept the worksheets she used in dialectical behavioral therapy (DBT) and sometimes reviews them, although "not like I probably should. I didn't like that therapy much. I don't freak out on people like the others I met. No distress tolerance," she announces, as if making a joke.

You ask if something happened today or recently that might have contributed to her feeling so low. She responds, drably, "Nothing out of the ordinary." She clears her throat and her voice seems more assured. Then you hear her yell to someone in her home, "I'm on the phone!" She then says to you, "I'll be there on Monday. Thank you for calling me, it means a lot."

DECISION POINT B

Given what you know about this patient so far, how should you address her risk for suicide? Points awarded for correct and incorrect answers are scaled from best (+5) to unhelpful but not harmful (0) to dangerous (−5).

B1. _____ The patient admits that she was suicidal just hours before you spoke. She now denies feeling suicidal but you are not comfortable with her "flight to health" and instruct her to go to the local psychiatric emergency room for an evaluation.

B2. _____ The patient admits that she was suicidal just hours before you spoke. She now denies feeling suicidal but you are not comfortable with her "flight to health" and instruct her to meet you at the local psychiatric inpatient unit where you have admitting privileges.

B3. _____ The patient admits that she was suicidal just hours before you spoke. She says she spent a year doing DBT where she learned how to cope with these feelings, but that was a year ago and in the moment she forgot many of the skills she typically uses in these situations. She now denies feeling suicidal and offers a safety plan that includes calling the emergency department and having family members close by. She mentions coping skills that include taking a shower, listening to music, reading in her backyard, or writing in her journal. You have

an appointment with her in 3 days' time. You conclude she is safe and tell her you look forward to meeting her on Monday.

B4. _____ The patient admits that she was suicidal just hours before you spoke. She says she spent a year doing DBT where she learned how to cope with these feelings, but that was a year ago and in the moment she forgot many of the skills she typically uses in these situations. She now denies feeling suicidal and offers a safety plan that includes calling the emergency department and having family members close by. She mentions coping skills that include taking a shower, listening to music, reading in her backyard, or writing in her journal. She carries a primary diagnosis of borderline personality disorder, so you conclude that a visit to the emergency room would further complicate her ability to recover by encouraging reliance upon an institution to solve her problems. You conclude she is safe and tell her you look forward to meeting her on Monday.

B5. _____ The patient admits that she was suicidal just hours before you spoke. She now denies feeling suicidal but you are not comfortable with her "flight to health" and instruct her to meet you at your office immediately so you can assess her for safety.

VIGNETTE PART 3

The patient arrives for her appointment as scheduled, dressed casually in jeans and a button-down long-sleeved shirt. She averts her gaze, limply shakes your hand, and then sits with her legs folded underneath her body on the chair opposite you. Her long brown hair appears poorly kempt and is partially covering her face. You welcome her to your office and tell her you are glad she decided to come. For several minutes she does not say anything. You wait. "I hate this part," she says at last. "Starting over with a new doctor," she begins. "I'm sick of telling my story because no one believes me." She reaches for a tissue from the box on the table. "I don't even know what I'm supposed to feel like anymore. All I know is that I hate this." Her voice thickens. "I'm on 450 mg of Effexor for depression, 200 mg of Seroquel for sleep—which does not work for me, by the way— and when my last doctor wanted to put me back on Depakote I started to cry, so I . . . ." You are unable to understand the rest of her sentence. She blows her nose. "I'm so sorry about this. You don't know me and I'm already crying like a baby."

You tell her that your office is a safe place for her to cry or express any emotion she feels. You remind her that everything you talk about together is confidential unless she says she wants to harm someone in which case you would be obligated to break confidentiality. She smiles and pulls her hair from her face. She is not wearing makeup, and her eyes are bloodshot from crying. You tell her you would like to get to know her better and determine how you can help. You explain that you prefer to organize the interview somewhat because the session is limited to 45 minutes, but that you will need two to three sessions to make your evaluation and that will give her a chance to see if she feels you are a good match for her.

She describes her depression as "feeling hopeless, helpless, worthless. I can't concentrate to save my life, my mind is constantly rolling over things I can't do anything about. I either eat too much or not at all, and I'm bored by things I know I should enjoy, like meeting people, going to a movie, gardening." She shakes her head. "I can't even garden! My brother is such an idiot! I spent all this time making a little vegetable garden in the backyard and he and his burn-out friends just ran through it playing Frisbee." She tells you that she cannot speak with anyone in her family. "My father says I'm faking everything. My mother is an alcoholic, so she's usually passed out in their bedroom. She has cancer, by the way. Even the dog hates me." She chuckles to herself. "Even the stupid dog!"

You ask when she began to feel depressed and she says, "I remember the exact moment everything changed." She tells you she was married for 2 years but they divorced 3 years ago. She met him at the bank where she currently works as a teller. "I've been a teller for 5 years and they will not promote me, but that is another story. I think it is to keep me from getting full benefits since they know I'm sick." She says the marriage started out "okay" and she was happy just getting out of her family's house. "Maybe that is why I married him, I don't know." In the past she had several close girlfriends, but they have drifted apart. She has had passive suicidal ideation "off and on" for the past 3 years, but never made an attempt and says she would never have the guts to do it. She does have a history of self-injurious behavior that began at the same time, including cutting her arm with a razor and punching her thigh until she has black and blue marks. The last time she hurt herself was Friday before you spoke. "I punched myself. Then I felt better. Then I wanted to do it again so I called."

She tells you she has been on too many medications and that "nothing works." Her past medication trials have included fluoxetine up to 80 mg, escitalopram up to 40 mg, bupropion up to 450 mg, nortriptyline up to 150 mg, augmentation strategies with valproic acid up to 1500 mg, lithium up to 450 mg b.i.d., quetiapine up to 200 mg, risperidone up to 3 mg, lorazepam up to 2 mg, clonazepam up to 2 mg, and zolpidem up to 10 mg. She remembers being on fluoxetine for about 1.5 years and felt better for only the first 2–3 months. Then her doctor kept raising the dose. Then he augmented first with bupropion, then valproic acid, then changed the valproic acid to lithium. She changed doctors because the valproic acid caused her to put on about 40 pounds and she became sick and tremulous on the lithium, so that was discontinued. The fluoxetine was discontinued by her second psychiatrist who started risperidone as a monotherapy. She

started at risperidone 0.5 mg b.i.d. and was quickly titrated to 1.5 mg b.i.d. over 2 weeks. She said she felt so tired she could not leave her room.

She stopped taking the risperidone because of the somnolence and when she told her new psychiatrist she "acted angry. She said if I was not going to take my medications she could not treat me. She told me I was borderline. I barely knew this doctor so I figured this was not a good match so I found my third shrink." The last psychiatrist started the patient on nortriptyline, which helped improve her mood for about 3 months. "That seems like my limit. After 3 months nothing works. I don't understand that. I have had these long bouts of depression that seem to last forever. Then I start to feel better, but then it happens again." She complains that her insomnia started around the same time as starting fluoxetine. "I had trouble sleeping before that, taking hours to fall asleep or waking several times through the night. Once I started Prozac, I could not sleep well at all. I've tried Benadryl, Trazodone, and Ambien. Some of the other drugs were supposed to help me sleep, too, but it seems like once this problem began, I can't get rid of it. I don't remember having a good solid night's sleep in 3 years. I know I used to sleep well when I was younger."

You ask what happened 3 years ago. She tells you that was when she was diagnosed with myasthenia gravis (MG). She gives you the name of her neurologist, her phone number, and signs permission for you to share medical information with her. She had noticed right before she got married that she was starting to have difficulty sustaining her energy, her legs would get weak, and sometimes her eyesight would become blurry, and she blamed it on stress. At their wedding, she tells you, she was having difficulty speaking and swallowing. She thought it was because she was nervous about the wedding but found she really could not swallow. She asked her ex-husband if she could trade her plate of food for his soup so she could eat something and he refused. "That is when I started seeing how cruel he could be."

She reaches for more tissues. "It just got worse," she explains. "I went to the doctor and after a bunch of tests they told me I had MG. I told my ex and do you know what he did? He had a gun and put it to his head." She shapes her hand like a pistol and points it at her temple. "He said he was going to kill himself if I did not stop lying to him. Lying? Why would I lie about having MG? Then he pointed the gun at me and I ran out of the house. That was the only time my father actually came over to our apartment. He picked me up and took me home. But he did not say a word the entire time. Like I was causing him some huge problem. Gee, Dad, I'm sorry I'm sick! I'm sorry my husband pulled a gun on me after threatening to kill himself. It is all my fault. I'm sorry I have to get IV treatments every weekend. I'm sorry my medications are so-o-o-o expensive. I should just die already. What use is it to go through all this treatment if nothing matters?" She bangs her fists on the armrests of her chair.

"I'm so sick of this!" She is inconsolable for a few minutes then calms down. "They want to fire me at work all the time. I know it is because they do not want to pay my insurance or let me go to doctor's appointments, which I have every week. The bitch that sits next to me keeps a heater on all the time and she just does not get it that it makes me feel worse." She complains that she feels depressed most of the time and finds it difficult to speak with her coworkers as she thinks they believe she is "faking her MG" to get special treatment at work. I don't have to be in early to open up, but I do stay late. I don't think my fellow tellers realize that is not a benefit!"

You ask what medications she takes for her MG. She responds that she takes cyclosporine and has weekly intravenous immunoglobulin (IVIG) treatments. She has had three inpatient treatments with high-dose steroids and was treated with prednisone for about 3 months but had to stop because she could not tolerate the medication. "I know not to drink grapefruit juice since I take cyclosporine, so don't worry about that."

DECISION POINT C

Given what you know about this patient, what is your differential diagnosis? +2 points given for correct answers, including rule-outs. −2 points are given for incorrect answers.

AXIS I:	
AXIS II:	
AXIS III:	

DECISION POINT D

Which of the patient's diagnoses would you consider to be her primary diagnosis? +5 points for correct answer. 0 points for incorrect answer.

D1. _____ Major depression
D2. _____ Dysthymia
D3. _____ Mood disorder secondary to a general medical condition
D4. _____ Myasthenia gravis
D5. _____ Other substance-induced mood disorder
D6. _____ Mental disorder not otherwise specified due to a general medical condition
D7. _____ Borderline personality disorder
D8. _____ Panic disorder without agoraphobia

DECISION POINT E

Given the patient's medication history, 1 year's worth of DBT, and the apparent resistance of her depressive symptoms to these interventions, how would you proceed with your evaluation? Points awarded for correct and incorrect answers are scaled from best (+5) to unhelpful but not harmful (0) to dangerous (−5).

E1. _____ Obtain laboratory results of her complete blood count (CBC), liver function tests, basic metabolic panel, thyroid function panel, and cholesterol panel, and check urine toxicology.
E2. _____ Get permission to speak with her neurologist about her treatment for MG.
E3. _____ Research the psychiatric side effects of MG and the treatment she is receiving for MG. Determine what psychiatric medications would be

contraindicated to use in conjunction with MG treatment.
E4. _____ Ask the patient about her understanding of MG and what daily life is like for her given this illness.
E5. _____ She has not tried a monoamine oxidase inhibitor (MAOI). Start the selegiline patch immediately, as it will take 4–6 weeks to reach therapeutic levels.
E6. _____ She is at high risk for suicide and resistant to pharmacotherapy. Begin electroconvulsive therapy (ECT) treatments to achieve remission of symptoms as quickly as possible, followed by either maintenance ECT if warranted or continued pharmacotherapy.
E7. _____ Try a combination of cognitive behavior therapy (CBT) or interpersonal psychotherapy (IPT) with psychopharmacological intervention.
E8. _____ Ask for permission to speak with family members.
E9. _____ Consider a day treatment program or a partial program.
E10. _____ Ask for permission to speak with former psychiatric treating clinicians.

ANSWERS: SCORING, RELATIVE WEIGHTS, AND COMMENTS

High positive scores (+3 and above) indicate a decision that would be effective, would be required for diagnosis, and without which management would be negligent. Lower positive scores (+2) indicate a decision that is important but not immediately necessary. The lowest positive score (+1) indicates a decision that is potentially useful for diagnosis and treatment. A neutral score (0) indicates a decision that is neither helpful nor harmful under the given circumstances. High negative scores (−5 to −3) indicate a decision that is inappropriate and potentially harmful or possibly life-threatening. Loser negative scores (−2 and above) indicate a decision that is nonproductive and potentially harmful.

DECISION POINT A

A1. ____ −5 This answer suggests a preconceived notion about the negative attributes of a patient with borderline personality disorder before you adequately evaluate the patient or establish a therapeutic relationship. You should keep an open mind about her diagnoses and assess her yourself before making quick judgments, especially if your countertransference toward patients with this presumed disorder will compromise your ability to treat her.

A2. ____ +2 This is true. You have not established a doctor-patient relationship with this woman and you are under no obligation to "begin treatment" by making a telephone call, whether it is 9 p.m. or any other time of day or night. She did make it clear by her second message that she will come to her appointment on Monday.

A3. ____ −5 Despite being correct about not being obliged professionally or ethically to engage this patient before establishing a doctor-patient relationship, as well as acknowledging that she has made it clear that her crisis has passed and she will come to the appointment on Monday, the final statement about her diagnosis of borderline personality disorder and your subsequent preconceived notion about how to deal with such patients suggests you would not give her appropriate and yet-to-be-determined care once she does arrive in your office.

A4. ____ +3 The decision to call back a patient who has not established a doctor-patient relationship with you, but was referred to you and is in apparent distress, endorsing suicidal ideation, is appropriate but, from a medico-legal perspective, not a requirement. Work done by Linehan, Rathus, and Miller suggests that the use of the telephone for coaching purposes, with chronically suicidal patients who have poor coping skills, who are engaged in DBT, and are in a crisis state, can be useful despite the paucity of evidence that it is necessary. They also contend that these patients tend not to abuse the privilege of using the telephone but find comfort knowing they could reach their therapist if they feel desperate.

A5. ____ +3 See answer for A4. In the absence of clear and replicated evidence that this improved some measurable outcome, the answer would receive more points.

DECISION POINT B

B1. ____ +3 It is almost always recommended that a patient be sent to the emergency room if you fear the patient may still be suicidal. In this case you certainly can address her risk of suicide over the telephone, but this answer suggests that you are not completely comfortable with her "flight to health" and feel that she is still at risk. A better answer would include asking whether there are any other family members, friends, or social supports who could be called to check on the patient immediately. Additionally, you should evaluate whether the patient is able to bring herself to the emergency room or whether you should send emergency medical services to pick her up.

B2. ____ +3 See answer for B1. Whether you have admitting privileges at the nearest emergency room is immaterial to her safety.

B3. ____ +4 You have assessed the patient over the phone and concluded that she can keep herself safe and has well-thought-out plans for maintaining that safety, and you have a follow-up plan to see her. She should be reassessed, however, the next day, especially if you do not know the patient well. A suggestion to call you or to call the local emergency room or crisis line to call the next day would be appropriate, assuming you would be available for follow up on this plan.

B4. ____ −5 Although the evaluation and plan seem perfectly reasonable and you are confident in the patient's ability to remain safe, you made the mistake of reacting to your preconceived notions of a patient for whom another clinician diagnosed borderline personality disorder. Your job as the new treating clinician, assuming you accept this patient into your practice once you meet her, is to perform your own complete evaluation and diagnose according to your own impressions. A great disservice is done to patients who have been labeled with certain especially stigmatized illnesses such as borderline personality disorder by subsequent doctors who blindly accept the diagnosis, are influenced by its perceived negative attributes, and begin a doctor-patient relationship with prejudice.

B5. ____ −5 You do not know this patient. If you do not feel she is safe, it is appropriate to assess her in person. However, this should be done in an emergency department for both the patient's protection and for your protection. You are not required to be the psychiatrist who assesses her. She has not given you the impression that she is

psychotic, but there have been cases of doctors being assaulted or even killed by psychotic patients who were seen in an emergency situation in a private office.

DECISION POINT C

AXIS I:	(+2) Major Depressive Disorder, Recurrent, Severe, without Psychotic Features (−2) Dysthymic Disorder (−2) Mood Disorder Secondary to a General Medical Condition; (−2) Other Substance Induced Mood Disorder; (−2) Mental Disorder Not Otherwide Specified Due to a General Medical Condition (−2) Panic Disorder without Agoraphobia
AXIS II:	(−2) Borderline Personality Disorder
AXIS III:	(+2) Myasthenia Gravis

Major Depressive Disorder, Recurrent, Severe, without Psychotic Features (+2). The patient meets the criteria, having depressed mood and anhedonia, explaining that she is bored by things she normally enjoys doing. She complains of poor mood most of the time, disturbed sleep, fatigue, feelings of hopelessness, helplessness, worthlessness, difficulty at work, and recurrent suicidal ideation. Her worry that co-workers consider her to be "faking" an illness to get special treatment was not fully explored as a paranoid delusion as she does leave work weekly, is excused from arriving at work early, staying late instead, and she does not express any other psychotic symptoms.

Dysthymic Disorder (−2). The patient does report feeling depressed more often than not, but has had remission of symptoms each year lasting up to 3 months at a time. Subsequently she does not meet the criteria for dysthymic disorder, which requires depressive symptoms more often than not for a consecutive period of 2 years.

Mood Disorder Secondary to a General Medical Condition (−2). There is sparse literature regarding psychiatric manifestations related directly to MG. It is likely the major depressive symptoms experienced by the patient are not the direct result of the physiological illness but rather the experience of the illness, ruling out this diagnosis.

Other Substance Induced Mood Disorder (−2). The medications the patient takes for MG include cyclosporine and weekly IVIG treatments. IVIG can cause anxiety, chills, dizziness, drowsiness, fatigue, fever, headache, irritability, lethargy, malaise, and aseptic meningitis syndrome. Some researchers have linked it specifically to depressive symptoms, especially when it is used as a treatment for cytokine-induced illness. Cyclosporine by itself is not known to cause psychiatric side effects. In the past the patient has received pulses of high-dose steroids and spent approximately 3 months taking prednisone, which she stopped because she was not able to tolerate it. It is well known that the use of steroids can cause psychosis and mood dysphoria. However, she is not taking these medications and has not taken them in awhile, and there is little evidence of these psychiatric side effects lasting after the dis-

continuation of the medication. One cannot, of course, rule out this possibility.

Mental Disorder Not Otherwise Specified Due to a General Medical Condition (−2). This diagnosis is reserved for situations in which the psychiatric symptoms are directly related to physiological effects of the medical condition, but the criteria are not met for a specific mental disorder due to a general medical condition. A direct link between the physiological effects of MG and psychiatric manifestations has not been adequately established.

Panic Disorder without Agoraphobia (−2). The patient has not given any information that would lead you to this diagnosis. You should explore the history of this diagnosis, however, in future sessions to determine whether the patient had panic attacks in the past and if she would require continued antidepressant medication that would address this diagnosis.

Borderline Personality Disorder (−2). This patient has unstable interpersonal relationships with coworkers and with her family. She gave no indication that she felt this way before the onset of her MG. Additionally, she does not display frantic efforts to avoid real or imagined abandonment, her interpersonal relationships are not characterized by alternating extremes of idealization and devaluation, she has not demonstrated or indicated she has an unstable self-image or sense of self, and she does not display affective instability. She does have recurrent suicidal ideation, not behaviors, she is impulsive in her maladaptive coping behavior of selfharm, does have chronic feelings of emptiness and seems to have a great deal of anger and possibly stress-related paranoid ideation. However, the feelings of emptiness, anger, and possible paranoia all can be traced to discernable and understandably reasonable psychosocial stressors. Her anger is not disproportionate or inappropriate, and she has worked at the same job for 5 years, indicating her behavior at work is probably not considered intolerable. The reasons for the bank not promoting her may have nothing to do with her psychiatric symptoms or personality structure. Finally, the symptoms that caused previous clinicians to label this patient as having borderline personality disorder may have been more severe in the past, but your present evaluation does not suggest an axis II diagnosis, but rather the sometimes maladaptive, but otherwise seemingly appropriate reaction to psychosocial and personal stressors relating to her medical illness.

Myasthenia Gravis(+2): True; this is her medical diagnosis and belongs in axis III.

DECISION POINT D

D1. _____ (+5) Major depression. See answers for Decision Point C. She does have a primary neurological illness, myasthenia gravis, and this is very likely the precipitant for her mood symptoms. However, in the context of a psychiatric evaluation, her primary diagnosis is major depression, recurrent, severe, without psychotic features.

DECISION POINT E

E1. _____ (+5) Before making a decision about pharmacotherapy, and especially because this patient has been taking medications that have harmful effects on liver, kidney, and thyroid function, as well as a risk for metabolic syndrome, it is prudent to get baseline laboratory values to better inform your decisions. Additionally, it is important to rule out other medical conditions that may be causing the depression, such as anemia, occult malignancy, hypothyroidism, or substance abuse.

E2. _____ (+5) It is good practice to coordinate care with other treating clinicians, especially those who are concurrently treating a major medical condition. You and the other clinicians will be better informed about the conditions each is treating, and establishment of such collaborative relationships will enhance the overall treatment of the patient.

E3. _____ (+5) This patient has a major neurological condition. If you do not already have expertise in the area of MG, a better understanding of the illness will enhance your informed decisions regarding the psychiatric issues you are treating. Finally, although the treatment with steroids stopped 3 months before you met the patient, the medication could have had an impact on her condition. For all of these reasons, close collaboration with her neurologist and obtaining as much collateral information as possible will help you in your diagnosis and treatment.

E4. _____ (+5) Exploring the patient's understanding of her MG, as well as her day-to-day experience coping with this illness, will better inform your psychiatric evaluation and understanding of the patient's daily life experiences.

E5. _____ (−5) She is taking venlafaxine and quetiapine. Trying an MAOI is a reasonable choice given that she has not done well when taking numerous other classes of antidepressants, mood stabilizers, and neuroleptic medications, and the MAOIs are indicated for treatment-resistant major depression. However, before starting an MAOI she must be weaned slowly from venlafaxine as its half-life of 5 hours along with the 11-hour half-life of its metabolite, *O*-desmethylvenlafaxine, causes a withdrawal syndrome. Venlafaxine is contraindicated for concurrent use with MAOIs because of the risk of serotonin syndrome (hypertension, hyperthermia, myoclonus, tremor, diarrhea, and mental status changes), so the transition must follow a washout period of 5 times the drug's half-life or at least 2 weeks (5 weeks if transitioning from fluoxetine, whose half-life is 84 hours or 7 days if its metabolites are included). This patient was taking venlafaxine 450 mg, which is twice the recommended upper-end dose. There is little evidence that this medication is more effective at more than 225 mg daily. Moreover, this patient has a greater likelihood of achieving remission of symptoms with ECT as treatment-refractory severe major depression is a clear indication for such treatment, long before so many medications were tried.

E6. _____ (+5) If the patient is willing, ECT is entirely appropriate, is clearly indicated, and could have been tried earlier than at this stage of her treatment, given her poor response to all other medication trials. It has also been demonstrated that muscle relaxants and ECT premedications can safely be given to patients with MG with appropriate precautions. Many argue that ECT should be tried after as few as two "failed" antidepressant trials. This patient has taken numerous antidepressants including selective serotonin reuptake inhibitors, serotonin-norepinephrine reuptake inhibitors, an atypical antidepressant (bupropion), and tricyclic antidepressants, as well as atypical neuroleptics, two mood stabilizers, and an assortment of benzodiazepines and hypnotics. The response rate to ECT is generally accepted as being in the 70%–90% range in patients who have not already demonstrated such resistance to pharmacotherapy, and it is efficacious in 15%–20% of pharmacotherapy treatment-resistant patients. Antidepressants generally will lead to full remission of symptoms in 50% of patients with treatment at an adequate dose for at least 6 weeks, 10%–15% will show some improvement, and the remainder will have little to no improvement of symptoms. Although ECT is not indicated for treatment of personality disorders, borderline personality disorder has not been clearly established and may have spuriously been diagnosed. The severity of her mood symptoms warrants immediate action.

E7. ____ (+5) Although there is an increasing number of studies indicating the effectiveness of IPT for depression (in this case, the patient's interpersonal relationships seem to be worsening her symptoms of depression since she became sick with MG) and CBT, especially when combined with psychopharmacological interventions, the gravity and duration of her severe symptoms suggest the need for immediate intervention, such as ECT. Once the severe symptoms have remitted, beginning psychotherapy such as IPT or CBT in conjunction with a pharmacological intervention such as an MAOI (given the history of her poor response to other classes of medications) may be appropriate for maintenance, and many studies indicate that this approach is more effective than pharmacotherapy alone.

E8. ____ (+5) The patient gave permission to call the neurologist and provided contact information. This will help you to firmly establish the diagnosis of MG, determine the medications the neurologist is using, and work collaboratively to help the patient's psychiatric issues. Further background obtained from family will help shed light on any prior psychiatric condition that may have existed on its own or become manifest because of the neurological condition of MG. Additionally, a family meeting will help you better understand the function of this family system and its potential for being supportive to the patient. The patient, of course, would have to consent to your speaking with her parents, with whom she clearly has a difficult relationship. You want to preserve your therapeutic working relationship and at the same time gather as much collateral information about the patient as is possible. Your approach to asking the patient's permission will therefore need to be empathic toward her difficulties with her family, but clear about the medical benefits from your being able to discuss hers and her family's history.

E9. ____ (+5) Given the difficulty the patient has with continuing work and the fact that she seems to be doing so to keep her insurance active, an exploration with the help of a social worker into a part-time or day hospitalization program until she is more stable may help this patient recover and more rapidly obtain additional services if such are available to her in her area.

E10. ____ (+5) Absolutely. You cannot proceed in this case without first speaking with as many of her previous clinicians as you can to determine why medications were chosen, how long they were used before something else was tried, what were the criteria for moving between agents, what were the results of each trial, why were so many medications tried before ECT was considered, and where did the diagnosis of borderline personality disorder come from. The other clinicians will provide invaluable information in a complicated case such as this.

SCORING

Decision Point	Score	Ideal Score
A		8
B		10
C		4
D		5
E		45
Total		72

KEY CLINICAL POINTS

1. It is essential not to allow prejudice, or preconceived ideas about a patient or their historic diagnosis to cause you to make poor clinical decisions.
2. If you do not know a patient who calls you expressing suicidal ideation, the safest way to assess for safety is face-to-face, in an emergency room.
3. A primary neurological illness may precipitate a psychiatric illness, or psychiatric illness may be a symptom of neurological illness, in either case the psychiatric illness must be treated.

REFERENCES

American Psychiatric Association: Practice guideline for the treatment of patients with major depressive disorder (3rd ed). Am J Psychiatry 2010; www.psych.org/guidelines/mdd2010

American Psychiatric Association: Practice guideline for the assessment and treatment of patients with suicidal behaviors. Am J Psychiatry 2003; 160(suppl 11):1–60

Calarge CA, Crowe RR: Electroconvulsive therapy in myasthenia gravis. Ann Clin Psychiatry 2004; 16:225–227

de Jonghe F, Hendricksen M, van Aalst G, Kool S, Peen V, Van R, van den Eijnden E, Dekker J: Psychotherapy alone and combined with pharmacotherapy in the treatment of depression. Br J Psychiatry 2004; 185:37–45

de Jonghe F, Kool S, van Aalst G, Dekker J, Peen J: Combining psychotherapy and antidepressants in the treatment of depression. J Affect Disord 2001; 64:217–229

de Mello MF, de Jesus Mari J, Bacaltchuk J, Verdeli H, Neugebauer R: A systematic review of research findings on the efficacy of interpersonal therapy for depressive disorders. Eur Arch Psychiatry Clin Neurosci 2005; 255:75–82

Doering S, Henze T, Schüssler G: Coping with myasthenia gravis and implications for psychotherapy. Arch Neurol 1993; 50:617–620

Fenton L, Fasula M, Ostroff R, Sanacora G: Can cognitive behavioral therapy reduce relapse rates of depression after ECT? A preliminary study. J ECT 2006; 22:196–198

Frank E, Kupfer DJ, Buysse DJ, Swartz HA, Pilkonis PA, Houck PR, Rucci P, Novick DM, Grochocinski VJ, Stapf DM: Randomized trial of weekly, twice-monthly, and monthly interpersonal psychotherapy as maintenance treatment for women with recurrent depression. Am J Psychiatry 2007; 164:761–767

Kelly MA, Cyranowski JM, Frank E: Sudden gains in interpersonal psychotherapy for depression. Behav Res Ther 2007; 45:2563–2572

Klein DN, Santiago NJ, Vivian D, Blalock JA, Kocsis JH, Markowitz JC, McCullough JP Jr, Rush AJ, Trivedi MH, Arnow BA, Dunner DL, Manber R, Rothbaum B, Thase ME, Keitner GI, Miller IW, Keller MB: Cognitive-behavioral analysis system of psychotherapy as a maintenance treatment for chronic depression. J Consult Clin Psychol 2004; 72:681–688

Kho KH, van Vreeswijk MF, Simpson S, Zwinderman AH: A meta-analysis of electroconvulsive therapy efficacy in depression. J ECT 2003; 19:139–147

Linehan MM, Comtois KA, Murray AM, Brown MZ, Gallop RJ, Heard HL, Korslund KE, Tutek DA, Reynolds SK, Lindenboim N: Two-year randomized controlled trial and follow-up of dialectical behavior therapy vs therapy by experts for suicidal behaviors and borderline personality disorder. Arch Gen Psychiatry 2006; 63:757–766

Paul RH, Cohen RA, Goldstein JM, Gilchrist JM: Severity of mood, self-evaluative, and vegetative symptoms of depression in myasthenia gravis. J Neuropsychiatry Clin Neurosci 2000; 12:499–501

Paykel ES, Scott J, Teasdale JD, Johnson AI, Garland A, Moore R, Jenaway A, Cornwall PL, Hayhurst H, Abbott R, Pope M: Prevention of relapse in residual depression by cognitive therapy: a controlled trial. Arch Gen Psychiatry 1999; 56:829–835

Prudic J, Sackeim HA, Devanand DP: Medication resistance and clinical response to electroconvulsive therapy. Psychiatry Res 1990; 31:287–296

Rush AJ, Trivedi MH, Wisniewski SR, Nierenberg AA, Stewart JW, Warden D, Niederehe G, Thase ME, Lavori PW, Lebowitz BD, McGrath PJ, Rosenbaum JF, Sackeim HA, Kupfer DJ, Luther J, Fava M: Acute and longer-term outcomes in depressed outpatients requiring one or several treatment steps: a Star*D report. Am J Psychiatry. 2006; 163:1905–1917

UK ECT Review Group: Efficacy and safety of electroconvulsive therapy in depressive disorders: a systematic review and meta-analysis. Lancet 2003; 361:799–808

Wampold BE, Minami T, Baskin TW, Callen TS: A meta-(re)analysis of the effects of cognitive therapy versus "other therapies" for depression. J Affect Disord 2002; 68:159–165

Yoshida K, Alagbe O, Wang X, Woolwine B, Thornbury M, Raison CL, Miller AH: Promoter polymorphisms of the interferon-α receptor gene and development of Interferon-induced depressive symptoms in patients with chronic hepatitis C: preliminary findings. Neuropsychobiology 2005; 52:55–61

A Keyed-Up Paper Chaser

VIGNETTE PART 1

Ms. P, a 24-year-old divorced law student, reluctantly goes to the local mental health clinic because she doesn't want to go to her school's mental health services for fear that she will see someone she knows. You have only 20 minutes before your next scheduled appointment. She is anxious and insists on seeing you even though you do not have time for a full evaluation, and she cannot come back today because of her class schedule. You agree to see her.

She complains of feeling "on edge" but not to the extent that she is in danger of failing out of law school. She reports that she has been having difficulty sleeping, especially over the past year, maybe two; she gets about 4–5 hours of broken sleep per night. She has tried in the past to have a couple of alcoholic drinks before bed but reports, "I don't like the feeling." A friend suggested she try smoking marijuana, which she said "calmed my nerves," but she says she no longer smokes pot because she heard that it affects short-term memory, which she cannot afford to lose given the demands of law school. Her parents both drink scotch and sodas every evening "to unwind," so the patient does not think that using alcohol or pot is "a big deal."

Ms. P was married immediately after high school for 1 year to her high school sweetheart, who was captain of the football team, but she complained that he was too jealous and did not want her to study with friends and often called her on her cell phone eight to ten times a day to check on her. She moved home after they separated, both to save money and because her parents "want me to be safe." She reports that her father works long hours and is away a lot. She describes her mother as "needy" and says, "She likes it when I'm around to help her with shopping or to have a lunch companion." She mentions that she was given Valium by one of her friends; it helped her sleep and relax, and she would like to know if it would be possible to get a prescription for it.

DECISION POINT A

Given this history, which of the following would you do? (Select as many as appropriate. Points are taken away for incorrect answers.)

A1. _____ Tell the patient that you understand she is under a great deal of stress but that 20 minutes is much too short a time to make an adequate assessment. Invite her to return to see you within 1 week for a full evaluation.

A2. _____ Tell the patient that you understand what she's going through since you were once a medical student and you know that law school is similarly stressful. Ask her how much Valium she took, prescribe a month's supply to help her when she's "on edge," and ask her to return to see you within a month for a full evaluation.

A3. _____ Ask her about her drinking and drug history. If she reports that she is drinking or using substances regularly, suggest an independent substance use evaluation.

A4. _____ Arrange an emergency psychiatric hospitalization.

A5. _____ Prescribe a week's supply of a selective serotonin reuptake inhibitor (SSRI) at a starting dose and tell her that it will help with her anxiety. Prescribe a minimal dose of a long-acting benzodiazepine to bridge the time before the SSRI reaches therapeutic efficacy. Tell her that she should come back to see you in 1 week so you can monitor her improvement.

DECISION POINT B

With what you have learned so far, what is your differential diagnosis? (Rank as many as appropriate, in order of their likelihood. Points are taken away for incorrect answers.)

B1. _____ It is too early to make any diagnoses
B2. _____ Substance-induced anxiety disorder
B3. _____ Major depressive episode
B4. _____ Bipolar II disorder
B5. _____ Social phobia
B6. _____ Panic disorder
B7. _____ Generalized anxiety disorder
B8. _____ Somatization disorder

VIGNETTE PART 2

Ms. P comes back to your clinic 2 weeks later for a scheduled appointment. She is particularly worried about her classes and concerned that she is not reading enough. She says that she sometimes becomes "paralyzed with fear" that she'll be called on in a class and not know the answer to a question, when her "rational side" knows she typically does know the answer. A couple of the members of her study group complained to her that she has become irritable lately and is sometimes difficult to work with. She noticed that when she is in her group her mind will go blank and she will not know what the conversation is about and require reminding. She has been experiencing this all year but says that it is getting worse. She and her classmates are applying for externships, and she is worried that she will not get "the one I deserve." She insists that she cannot work in any area of law but corporate law, because "that's what my father does" and she is not interested in any other area. She also knows that this is one of the most competitive areas.

On further investigation of her medical history, she self-effacingly complains that she has had diarrhea nearly constantly for 3 years, for which she has had at least two hospital admissions and has been seen by several gastrointestinal specialists, who have not been able to give her a definitive diagnosis despite a battery of invasive tests. She reports frequent headaches and has been evaluated by several neurologists, who have told her that she does not have a brain tumor or migraines. One of her cousins died of an astrocytoma, and two of her aunts have migraines.

DECISION POINT C

Does the new information change your differential diagnosis? (Rank as many as appropriate, in order of their likelihood. Points are taken away for incorrect answers.)

C1. _____ It is too early to make any diagnoses
C2. _____ Substance-induced anxiety disorder
C3. _____ Major depressive episode
C4. _____ Bipolar II disorder
C5. _____ Social phobia
C6. _____ Panic disorder
C7. _____ Generalized anxiety disorder
C8. _____ Somatization disorder

VIGNETTE PART 3

Ms. P says that in high school she was "popular," with lots of friends and several boyfriends, and she continues to have no difficulty making friends. She has a brand-new car that she says is a "lemon" because she has had it in the shop three times in 3 months for "odd sounds it should definitely not be making, and they can't find a thing wrong with it." Her father, a wealthy attorney, has mentioned that he had similar problems with some of his cars in the past, so he is not surprised, and he helps her by lending her a car when hers is in the shop. Her mother worries that Ms. P is overreacting to "the little things" and keeps asking her if she's using illegal drugs, which she denies. She has been single since her divorce because, she complains, "I don't have the energy to put up with somebody else's worries when I have enough of my own for two or three people."

DECISION POINT D

On the basis of this information, which of the following would you inquire about to make a diagnosis of generalized anxiety disorder? (Select as many as appropriate. Points are taken away for incorrect answers.)

D1. _____ Does she experience periods of restlessness? Does she feel "keyed up" or "on edge"?
D2. _____ Is she easily fatigued?
D3. _____ Has she been irritable?
D4. _____ Does she have racing thoughts?
D5. _____ Has she experienced chest pain or a feeling of "impending doom"?
D6. _____ Has she had a weight loss of more than 20 pounds in the past 3 months?
D7. _____ Does she have a family history of alcohol abuse or dependence?

DECISION POINT E

Which of the following would be appropriate interventions at this time? (Select as many as appropriate. Points are taken away for incorrect answers.)

E1. _____ Recommending cognitive behavior therapy once per week
E2. _____ Recommending long-term psychodynamic therapy
E3. _____ Prescribing clonazepam
E4. _____ Prescribing buspirone
E5. _____ Prescribing paroxetine
E6. _____ Prescribing venlafaxine
E7. _____ Referring the patient to a local chapter of Alcoholics Anonymous
E8. _____ Prescribing a low dose of divalproex
E9. _____ Suggesting that the patient exclude refined sugars from her diet

ANSWERS: SCORING, RELATIVE WEIGHTS, AND COMMENTS

High positive scores (+3 and above) indicate a decision that would be effective, would be required for diagnosis, and without which management would be negligent. Lower positive scores (+2) indicate a decision that is important but not immediately necessary. The lowest positive score (+1) indicate a decision that is potentially useful for diagnosis and treatment. Neutral scores (0) indicate a decision that is neither clearly helpful nor harmful under the given circumstances. High negative scores (−3) indicate a decision that is inappropriate and potentially harmful or possibly life-threatening. Lower negative scores (−2) indicate a decision that is nonproductive and potentially harmful. The lowest negative score (−1) indicates a decision that is not harmful but is nonproductive, time consuming, and not cost effective.

DECISION POINT A

A1. _____ +5 The length of this evaluation is too short and the information too incomplete to make an informed diagnosis. Asking her to come back would both allow for a more substantial evaluation and contribute to the creation of a therapeutic relationship.

A2. _____ −3 The opening statement may be empathetic and can help normalize and validate the patient's feelings of anxiety. However, given some of her character traits, she may interpret this as a lack of empathy. Prescribing a controlled substance on such minimal evidence, especially with hints of substance or alcohol abuse, is not advisable.

A3. _____ +3 This is necessary given the hints of the patient's willingness to self-medicate, especially with illegal drugs. The therapist must be careful of how this is phrased, so that the patient-physician relationship is not damaged and a therapeutic alliance can be forged. If the patient's history offered specific indications of abuse or dependence, substance or alcohol abuse/dependence rehabilitation should be considered.

A4. _____ −5 At this point a psychiatric hospitalization is unwarranted. There is no evidence of a psychiatric emergency, such as psychosis, a severe major depressive episode, suicidality, or mania. Trying to force an admission would disrupt the patient-physician relationship.

A5. _____ +1 SSRIs are safe but will take a while to be effective. Although it is usually not good practice to prescribe a medication with minimal evidence for diagnosis and no method of mon-

itoring the patient, starting such a relatively safe medication given this scenario could serve as a transitional object and help reinforce the patient's own need to return for further treatment.

DECISION POINT B

B1. _____ +3 (Add 2 points if this was your primary response on the differential.) Yes, there is not enough information to make an informed diagnosis. The information is suggestive of many psychiatric diagnoses but also suggestive of normal variants.

B2. _____ 0 It is too early to make this diagnosis. You first need to explore substance and alcohol use, since the patient hints that this may have been a problem. Additionally, she may have stopped using alcohol on her own.

B3. _____ −1 There is no evidence of a depressive disorder. Decreased sleep over a long period is a nonspecific finding, and there are no other symptoms indicative of this diagnosis.

B4. _____ −1 There is no evidence of bipolar II disorder. Decreased sleep over a long period is not evidence of a manic or hypomanic episode.

B5. _____ −1 There is no evidence for this diagnosis thus far.

B6. _____ 0 Her decision to move back with her parents could be a practical decision given her recent divorce, her demanding educational responsibilities, and other considerations. Currently in the United States it is not uncommon for college graduates to move back home with their families until they are better able to manage on their own, so this is not culturally aberrant. Additionally, there is no evidence of a pathological need on the part of the patient to stay home with her parents, such as agoraphobia, or a pervasive and excessive need to be taken care of that leads to submissive and clinging behavior and fears of separation, as in dependent personality disorder.

B7. _____ +1 There certainly is some evidence to support this diagnosis, but the differential is too great and the symptoms are still too nonspecific. The only symptoms that point more specifically toward GAD are her complaint that she is "on edge."

B8. _____ 0 The patient has no physical complaints up to this point.

DECISION POINT C

C1. _____ 0 There is enough evidence at this point to make a diagnosis, and waiting for more information, while usually helpful, is not necessary to begin treatment.

C2. _____ +1 There is enough evidence to suggest that alcohol or other substances are playing a role in the patient's life that may be a cause for her other psychiatric complaints—not enough to make a primary diagnosis, however. She does not endorse depressed mood but does complain of irritability. You would want to know more details about her alcohol use to clarify this issue.

C3. _____ −1 A diagnosis of major depressive episode requires either symptoms of loss of interest or pleasure and/or depressed mood.

C4. _____ −1 A diagnosis of bipolar II disorder requires the presence or history of one or more major depressive episodes, the presence or history of at least one hypomanic episode, and no evidence ever of a manic or mixed episode.

C5. _____ +1 Social phobia, also known as social anxiety disorder, should be specified as generalized or nongeneralized (specific to one type of situation). A social phobia features a marked and persistent fear of one or more social or performance situations in which the person is exposed to unfamiliar people or to possible scrutiny by others. The individual fears that he or she will act in a way (or show anxiety symptoms) that will be humiliating or embarrassing. Exposure to the feared social situation almost invariably provokes anxiety, which may take the form of a situationally bound or situationally predisposed panic attack. Ms. P has described anxiety symptoms related to school, namely, being called on in class and difficulties encountered in her study group.

C6. _____ −1 Panic disorder requires recurrent unexpected panic attacks, and at least one of the attacks must have been followed by 1 month or more of persistent concern about having additional attacks, worry about the implications or consequences of the attack, or a significant change in behavior related to the attack. A panic attack is a discrete period of intense fear or discomfort in which four or more of the following symptoms developed abruptly and reached a peak within 10 minutes: palpitations; pounding heart, or accelerated heart rate; sweating; trembling or shaking; sensations of shortness of breath or smothering; feeling of choking; chest pain or discomfort; nausea or abdominal distress; feeling dizzy, unsteady, lightheaded, or faint; derealization or depersonalization; fear of losing control or going crazy; fear of dying; paresthesias; and chills or hot flushes.

C7. _____ +5 (Add 2 points if this was your primary response on the differential.) Ms. P's worry about school performance occurred consistently for at least 6 months. She indicates that she had difficulty controlling her worries, attempted self-medication, and is now seeking help. She feels "on edge," has difficulty concentrating, has been irritable, complains that her mind goes blank, and reports a disturbance in her sleep. She does not describe the focus of her anxiety as confined to panic attacks or symptoms of social phobia as described above.

C8. _____ +1 While Ms. P does have a history of somatic complaints occurring before age 30 for which she sought treatment and which caused her significant impairment in function, for a diagnosis of somatization disorder she must also have four pain symptoms: two gastrointestinal symptoms, one sexual symptom, and one pseudoneurological symptom. Her complaints were not diagnosed as actual physiological problems by multiple specialists, but she does not give the impression that she is feigning her illnesses, nor is there evidence of secondary gain. Recall that she "self-effacingly" revealed this information only after additional investigation. Further history may reveal that she does have additional complaints, so this diagnosis can remain on the differential. Moreover, a person who has generalized anxiety disorder may also have additional diagnoses, especially other anxiety disorders.

DECISION POINT D

D1. _____ +3 Correct

D2. _____ +3 Correct

D3. _____ +3 Correct

D4. _____ −3 This is nonspecific and suggests an affective disorder, not an anxiety disorder.

D5. _____ −3 This suggests a panic attack or a myocardial infarction, not generalized anxiety disorder.

D6. _____ −3 This is not specific for generalized anxiety disorder.

D7. _____ −3 While substance abuse is a common comorbid condition, it is not needed to make the diagnosis of generalized anxiety disorder.

DECISION POINT E

E1. _____ +3 Cognitive therapy directly addresses the patient's cognitive distortions, and behavioral approaches address somatic symptoms and self-defeating behavior directly. There is evidence that the combination is more effective than either part alone. This particular patient would likely benefit from cognitive behavior therapy.

E2. _____ +1 If the patient can afford long-term psychodynamic therapy, this could help her explore the unconscious conflicts, whatever they are and whenever they appeared in the course of her development, that may be expressed as anxiety. This could be a good strategy for longer-term treatment, but it is not appropriate in the acute setting.

E3. _____ +3 Benzodiazepines have long been considered the drug of choice for generalized anxiety disorder. Additionally, there is the possibility of selecting medications with a shorter half-life and a quicker onset for acute crises or longer-acting formulations to provide more consistent coverage. However, 25%–30% of all patients do not respond to a benzodiazepine trial, and some patients develop tolerance and dependency. The choice of benzodiazepine should be based on potency, half-life, side effects, and the specific symptoms targeted.

E4. _____ +1 This is a potentially useful treatment if the patient does not require immediate relief of symptoms, since the drug requires 4–6 weeks to become effective. However, it does have fewer side effects than the benzodiazepines (e.g., drowsiness, psychomotor impairment, and alcohol potentiation), and it has less potential for abuse.

E5. _____ +3 SSRIs have been shown to have significant antianxiety effects, but they take 3–4 weeks to become effective and may transiently increase anxiety, especially fluoxetine. This is why paroxetine and sertraline are better choices. They are safe medications in general and are not known for abuse.

E6. _____ +3 Venlafaxine extended release has been approved for generalized anxiety disorder. Published studies have reported efficacy both in acute settings (Davidson et al. 1999; Rickels et al. 2000) and in 6-month continuation trials (Gelenberg et al. 2000).

E7. _____ −1 Unless there is evidence of alcohol abuse or dependence, this is inappropriate.

E8. _____ −1 There is no evidence supporting the use of mood stabilizers to treat generalized anxiety disorder.

E9. _____ 0 Some believe that high levels of sugar in the diet may increase anxiety, although the evidence is mostly anecdotal; reducing sugar intake should not be considered as a first-line treatment in the case of Ms. P.

YOUR TOTAL

Decision Point	Your Score	Ideal Best Score
A		9
B		6
C		10
D		9
E		14
Total		48

KEY CLINICAL POINTS

1. In the assessment of a patient presenting with anxiety, rule out both physical causes and substance abuse. These can mimic most anxiety disorders or exacerbate the patient's condition.
2. Mood disorders, frequently comorbid with anxiety should be high on your differential diagnosis list.
3. Cognitive behavioral therapy (CBT) has significant research backing its efficacy in the treatment of anxiety disorders.
4. Medications from several classes of psychopharmacological agents, benzodiazepines, serotonin reuptake inhibitors, serotonin-norepinephrine reuptake inhibitors, reduce symptoms of anxiety disorders. The physician must weigh the pros and cons of any medication before prescribing.

REFERENCES

Davidson JR: First-line pharmacotherapy approaches for generalized anxiety disorder. J Clin Psychiatry. 2009;70 Suppl 2:25–31

Davidson JR, DuPont RL, Hedges D, Haskins JT: Efficacy, safety, and tolerability of venlafaxine extended release and buspirone in outpatients with generalized anxiety disorder. J Clin Psychiatry 1999; 60:528–535

Gelenberg AJ, Lydiard RB, Rudolph RL, Aguiar L, Haskins JT, Salinas E: Efficacy of venlafaxine extended-release capsules in nondepressed outpatients with generalized anxiety disorder: a 6-month randomized controlled trial. JAMA 2000; 283:3082–3088

Hunot V, Churchill R, Teixeira V, Silva de Lima M. Psychological therapies for generalized anxiety disorder. *Cochrane Database of Systematic Reviews* 2007, Issue 1. Art. No.: CD001848. DOI: 10.1002/14651858.CD001848.pub4.

Kapczinski FFK, Silva de Lima M, dos Santos Souza JJSS, Batista Miralha da Cunha AABC, Schmitt RRS. Antidepressants for generalized anxiety disorder. *Cochrane Database of Systematic Reviews* 2003, Issue 2. Art. No.: CD003592. DOI: 10.1002/14651858.CD003592

Rickels K, Pollack MH, Sheehan DV, Haskins JT: Efficacy of extended-release venlafaxine in nondepressed outpatients with generalized anxiety disorder. Am J Psychiatry 2000; 157:968–974

Sadock BJ, Sadock VA: Synopsis of Psychiatry, 10th ed. Philadelphia, Lippincott Williams & Wilkins, 2007

Schatzberg AF, Nemeroff CB: Essentials of Clinical Psychopharmacology, 2nd Edition. Arlington, VA, American Psychiatric Publishing, 2006

6

Obsessive-Compulsive Disorder

I Cannot Get the Thought Out of My Head

VIGNETTE PART I

You are an adult psychiatrist in independent practice. You receive a phone message from a 24-year-old woman who is close to finishing her MBA at a competitive program in your city. She recently stopped seeing the psychiatrist she had been seeing for the past 2 years. She complains that she is not getting better and would like a second opinion. In her message, she sounds distressed and asks you to call her back to set up an appointment because, "I feel like I'm losing my mind. I need help." You ask her if she is currently thinking about hurting or killing herself or anyone else and she responds, "I do not want to kill myself—I know it is stupid—but I cannot get the thought out of my head. I get other thoughts; like I'm never going to be a good mother and until I pat my head five times, I'll keep thinking it. I even think about killing my children, which I don't have. I don't even date!" She says she can stay safe and her mother is with her. You make it clear that if she feels like she is in danger of hurting herself she should call the local emergency room immediately. She says, "I think I'll be okay" with her mother, a registered nurse, but she insists upon seeing you. You arrange an urgent appointment for that evening. She tells you her mother will bring her.

The patient arrives. She is dressed smartly, is well-groomed, and is very polite but does not offer her hand to you when you reach out to shake hers as an introduction. She inspects the chair toward which you direct her to sit, looks around your office for something, and then seems to force herself to sit down. You note that within minutes she begins picking at individual hairs and there is a small round spot behind her right ear where hair is missing. The patient is visibly distraught and before she starts to talk you see her eyes well with tears. You wait for a few minutes. She does not say anything, so you ask a few general, nonthreatening questions in an attempt to help her relax and build a rapport. She stops you and says, "Sometimes I forget I pull my hair. I've been doing this for years. Sometimes I can stop, but right now I cannot. I get into these fits of anxiety and this is the only thing that makes me feel better."

She tells you she has 2 months left to complete her MBA and she has had six job interviews scheduled over the last 4 months. She was not able to make it to any of them. "I bought two new interview suits, I practiced what I was going to say—all of this with my mother's help, mind you—but in the end I could not get myself to leave the house. Now I do not know what I'm going to do. I could not even pick between the two suits and my mother had to force me to buy them both because I kept her at the store for 3 hours. I don't think I can get these interviews back and I'm worried I may have ruined my career forever." She begins to sob and takes a tissue from her purse, ignoring the box you provided on the table beside her in plain view. "I could not even leave my house at all until today and that is only because I made this appointment with you."

Since starting undergraduate school she lived in the dorms with a roommate, then found an apartment with a different roommate during graduate school. She moved out of the apartment 6 months before finishing her MBA because of interpersonal trouble with her roommate and moved back home with her mother. She says her mother has been very helpful, but she can tell that her "problems" have begun to "drive my mother crazy, and it looks like I'm going to have to move out." Her sobbing intensifies. "I do not know how I can do this. I have no place else to go."

You ask her why things seem to be worse now. For a moment she stops sobbing and seems to be thinking. Then she says, "I've got OCD [obsessive-compulsive disorder]. I must have. And it is taking over my life." You ask her what she means by that. "I do not know if it is specifically OCD—I'm not a psychiatrist—but I know that I've been having these thoughts, they just jump into my head, some of them horrible and violent, and little things I used to think were just my silly superstitions are now the focus of my day." She tells you that as a child she had to be sure that her dolls were always in a particular order (shortest to tallest to shortest) on her bed, and that she would both remove them and replace them each day to use her bed in precisely the same manner. If she moved one doll by accident ahead of another, she would have to start all over or "it just did not feel right. I know it is stupid. Believe me, I know this is ridiculous." She laughs nervously. "Since I was a kid I would have to keep all of the food on my plate completely separated, and if one thing touched another, like the potatoes touching the green beans, I would cry and my mother would fix me a new plate." She looks at you. "My grandfather used to tell me, "it all goes to the same place!' But I always felt that if the food touched on the plate then it would cause me to do something bad in school. Is this the dumbest thing you ever heard?"

Her posture in the chair does not change. She takes each used tissue, carefully folds it and places each tissue in her purse. "I think I'm starting to have panic attacks, too." She describes her last episode as happening 4 weeks ago at the supermarket; she was with her mother. They were in the cereal aisle and someone had accidentally knocked a few boxes of cereal onto the floor. She remembers staring at the boxes and becoming sweaty, her heart started to pound, her palms were moist, she felt dizzy, nauseated, and like she was "losing her mind"; her chest hurt as if "someone was stabbing me." At the time she wondered if she were having a heart attack and told her mother she needed to go to the emergency room. Within 10 minutes the attack subsided, but she still took the ambulance ride to the hospital and was told that her heart was fine, but that she probably had a panic attack. There was no precipitant to the attack that she can think of. It came on "out of the blue."

"I haven't gone shopping since. I stay at home. I do not even want to go into the back yard to sit on the deck. I stay inside all day watching TV. Now I'm feeling depressed and hopeless. I feel like I can't go out or something bad is going to happen to me. I worry if I go out I'll have another attack and there will not be anyone to help me."

DECISION POINT A

Given what you have learned so far from this patient's presentation, do you believe she should be seen in the local psychiatric emergency room? Points awarded for correct and incorrect answers are scaled from best (+5) to unhelpful but not harmful (0) to dangerous (−5).

A1. _____ Yes, the patient has described feeling suicidal. At this point you do not have corroborative evidence from her mother about the patient or their relationship. She should go to the emergency room to be evaluated for safety.

A2. _____ Yes, the patient has described feeling suicidal and should be evaluated for safety. At this point you do not have corroborative evidence from her mother about the patient or their relationship. Additionally, you should give her alprazolam 1 mg from your stock of samples to treat her panic disorder.

A3. _____ No, the patient can be treated as an outpatient. You should give her alprazolam 1 mg from your stock of samples to treat her panic disorder and arrange for her to see a cognitive behavioral therapist as soon as possible.

A4. _____ Not at this time. She has a safety plan including her mother staying with her. You can manage this patient as an outpatient unless her symptoms further deteriorate, at which point you would admit her.

A5. _____ Not at this time. She should be further assessed, including a mental status examination; history and evaluation of any additional comorbid mental illnesses and her particular obsessions and compulsions; family history; and evaluation of her potential for self-harm or suicide, impulsivity, violent or aggressive behaviors.

VIGNETTE PART II

You obtain a more detailed psychiatric and medical history. The patient reports feeling depressed "off and on" since she was a junior in high school. She never received psychiatric treatment, but did go to her school's guidance counselor every 1–2 weeks to talk about issues when they came up. She has never taken psychiatric medications. Until recently, she never thought about dying or killing herself, and these thoughts are very distressing to her. "I'm not like this. I know I'm not. I always had friends. I was on the cheerleading squad at high school, I graduated from an Ivy League university with a 3.8, and I went to another prestigious university for my MBA." She does not recall ever going with little sleep yet feeling refreshed the next day. "I need my sleep," she smiles. She never used to get irritable, but over the past 6 months she noticed that she "snaps" very easily. She would like to work for a corporation because she prefers to be "one among many" rather than attempt to work in a smaller business or start her own. "At one time I wanted to work for one of the big investment houses in New York City, but now I can't imagine how I would be able to walk down the street with so many people." She started feeling as though people were watching her or noticing that she performs little rituals such as touching the top right corner of a doorway three times with the pad of her index finger before entering a room. "If I did it before entering a room, people would like me. If I did not, I was sure someone would hate me." She sighs, then tries to laugh. "I used to avoid cracks on the sidewalk like every other kid, but now I have trouble even walking down the street."

She denies any current use of tobacco, alcohol, or other substances, although there was a period during college when she was drinking to excess. She stopped when someone close to her died during a car accident, driving while intoxicated. When asked about whether she was ever abused, she says her uncle fondled her from age 12 to 14 and was eventually jailed. "That is why my parents split up. My father did not believe his brother would do what he did." She denies self-mutilating behaviors, aggressive or violent behaviors, and anorexia or bulimia nervosa but has experienced extreme mood swings, especially in the past 6 months.

She had her tonsils and adenoids removed when she was 3 years old, a mole removed at 12 years of age, mononucleosis for approximately 1 month during 9th grade, but no other medical problems. She never had head trauma, loss of consciousness, or seizures, and is taking no medications other than birth control pills.

Her father and mother separated when she was 13 and divorced when she was 15. She describes it as "ugly." In the end, her mother had full legal custody and her father "gave up." Because she was mad at her father for taking her uncle's side in the molestation case she did not speak with him until she was accepted to the university. Now they speak weekly; she sees him at least once per month but not in the past half-year because of her difficulties in leaving the house. Her mother will not allow him to come to her house.

Currently, she reports that she has difficulty initiating sleep and has frequent wakenings. She describes lying in bed ruminating about whether she completed all the tasks she writes out for herself every night, sometimes staying up late, simply making a long list. Normally, she is a "self-motivated" student who works "harder than most of my classmates." Some of her MBA project colleagues have told her she is difficult to work with and at times, "inflexible," but she disagrees with that assessment. "I like things to be done a certain way, but I'm able to be flexible." She is very well-organized in the way she does her work. "I love office supplies!" But she says most of her colleagues are like this because "you have to be in this program. A mess on your desk or in your room is an outward manifestation of an inner spiritual state." She sits back and lets you ponder what she seems to feel is a deep thought.

She is typically forward-thinking but recently, since her symptoms have "taken over," she has lost interest in trying to figure out what to do with her life. She feels as though she is responsible for the rituals and obsessive thinking and as a result is very hard on herself. She has increasingly diminished energy as she feels more helpless and hopeless and is unable to focus even on a TV show without being easily distracted. Her appetite is less than usual, but she has not had major changes of weight. During the interview, she has diminished kinetics, sitting still in her chair.

You tell her you have to end the session, but you would like her to come back in 2 days when you have your first open appointment. She agrees and says she feels a little better after having spoken with you.

DECISION POINT B

Given what you learned from the patient's presentation, what is your differential diagnosis? (+2) points are given for correct answers, including appropriate rule-out diagnoses, and (−2) points are given for incorrect answers.

AXIS I:	
AXIS II:	

DECISION POINT C

Which of the following statements are true and which are false? (+2) points for each correct answer.

C1. _____ Obsessions are intrusive, persistent, unwanted thoughts, impulses, or images that give rise to marked anxiety or distress.

C2. _____ There are several established environmental risk factors for OCD including exposure to authority figures such as teachers who have OCD, exposure to close friends, or romantic relationships with individuals who have OCD.

C3. _____ Higher rates of OCD symptom severity, such as higher rates of compulsions without obsessions and higher rates of clinically significant OCD symptoms, are associated with early-onset OCD.

C4. _____ The symptoms of OCD between children and adults are very different.

C5. _____ Streptococcal infection may be associated with a form of early-onset OCD, often abbreviated PANDAS (pediatric autoimmune neuropsychiatric disorder associated with streptococcal infection), that involves an abrupt onset of OCD symptoms and co-occurring tics.

C6. _____ The mean age of OCD onset ranges from 18 to 22 years of age, with at least one third of cases beginning by age 40.

C7. _____ The heritability of panic disorder is roughly 22%.

C8. _____ In two of the larger twin studies for OCD, concordance rates ranged from 80% to 87% for monozygotic twins and from 47% to 50% for dizygotic twins.

C9. _____ OCD can be caused by neurological conditions such as brain trauma, stroke, encephalitis, temporal lobe epilepsy, Prader-Willi syndrome, Sydenham's chorea, carbon monoxide poisoning, manganese poisoning, and neurodegenerative diseases such as Parkinson's disease and Huntington's disease.

C10. _____ A compulsion is a physical or mental act by the patient whose performance of this act is done to undo a thought, magically prevent a feared event, or reduce anxiety or distress.

VIGNETTE PART III

The patient goes home with her mother and returns for her scheduled appointment in 2 days. She still seems distressed but tells you she feels better since talking to you. You ask to speak with her mother for collateral information, to which the patient consents. The patient's mother reports that she noticed the behaviors the patient described, but adds that in the past 4–6 months the patient has also started checking door locks several times, turning off the sink three times each time

she uses it, and has had at least four panic attacks that she witnessed. She retells the story about the supermarket in an identical fashion to the patient's version.

She tells you the patient was born at 38 weeks with a normal vaginal delivery. The mother did not use medications during pregnancy, there were no complications, and the patient had APGAR scores of 9 and 9. The patient did not require a stay in the neonatal intensive care unit and was promptly discharged with her mother within 2 days. She described the patient's temperament as fussy, colicky, and anxious. She walked at 1 year, talked at 1 year, was potty trained at 2.5 years, and never had problems with separation anxiety. The patient did well in school until middle school when she was molested by her uncle. At that point her grades suffered for about 6 months; her mother found a child psychiatrist and the patient was seen for psychotherapy over the next 3 years, partly due to the molestation and the cantankerous divorce. "She has a way of blocking things out. I quit trying." After that, her mother tells you, "she seemed to be back to normal, whatever that means. She received straight A's at a competitive school and I did not think there was a problem until recently." Her mother does not recall any episodes of her daughter having insomnia, grandiosity, hyperverbal or pressured speech, or risky behaviors. "She has always been an angel, a very thoughtful person." She goes on: "Her last psychiatrist wanted to give her medication after medication until she told me she "could not feel anything' anymore, or she was having severe stomach aches and headaches. We asked the doctor to take her off the medications and then we never went back."

Her daughter's mood has been increasingly low, and this is worrisome to the patient's mother. "She normally likes to garden with me, go to an occasional movie on the weekend, go out to dinner, or spend time with her friends. I do not think she has talked to her friends in months. When they call, she tells me to say she is not at home."She tells you her daughter mentioned feeling like she wanted to die a few times over the past month; she feels so frustrated spending so much time doing little rituals or not being able to stop thinking about something." They have had conversations about drugs and alcohol and the patient's mother does not keep any alcohol in the house. Two months ago she locked her own medications in a drawer because she did not want "to take a chance her daughter might do something stupid."

You ask about the family's psychiatric history. On the mother's side there are two cousins in their 40s with major depressive disorder who are in treatment and doing well. On the father's side, there is alcoholism in her father (sober for 14 years) and uncle (alcoholic, now in prison), and possible schizophrenia in two great-uncles.

The patient returns and both the patient and her mother would like to discuss treatment options. "I'm desperate, Doctor," says the patient. "I'll do anything you say. I cannot live like this."

You ask her to complete a Y-BOCS (Yale-Brown Obsessive Compulsive Scale) and she scores 27 out of 40, indicating severe symptoms.

DECISION POINT D

Given what you know about this patient and her history, how would you treat this patient? Answers are true or false. (+2) points for correct answers and (−2) points for incorrect answers.

D1. _____ First, you must establish a therapeutic alliance.

D2. _____ You already know enough about the patient's symptoms to make a correct diagnosis of OCD and Panic Disorder with Agoraphobia. Tell the patient you will start therapy with an selective serotonin reuptake inhibitor (SSRI) plus refer her to a cognitive behavioral therapist. You ask to see her again in 3 months to monitor her medications.

D3. _____ Further explore all of the patient's symptoms.

You do not know her well and you have already noted that her mother has additional collateral information the patient did not reveal. Differentiate her symptoms from other psychiatric disorders that have similar symptomatology, such as depressive ruminations, generalized anxiety disorder, intrusive thoughts and images of posttraumatic stress disorder, and schizophrenic and manic delusions.

D4. _____ Evaluate the patient's safety to protect against self-harm or harming others.

D5. _____ Complete the psychiatric assessment.

D6. _____ Establish goals for treatment.

D7. _____ Establish the appropriate setting for treatment.

D8. _____ Enhance treatment adherence.

DECISION POINT E

What would you choose as your initial treatment modality? Points range from (+5) points for the best answer to (−5) points for dangerous.

E1. _____ Cognitive behavioral therapy (CBT) with exposure and response prevention (ERP) only

E2. _____ CBT with ERP plus a serotonin response inhibitor (SRI)

E3. _____ An SRI alone

E4. _____ An SRI augmented with clomipramine

E5. _____ Clomipramine augmented with an SRI

ANSWERS: SCORING, RELATIVE WEIGHTS, AND COMMENTS

DECISION POINT A

A1. _____ +5 The patient describes feeling suicidal but has not divulged any intention or plan. She is ambivalent about her ability to remain safe at present. You should definitely explore her feelings about suicide and determine how safe she is to make a decision about a trip to the emergency room and potentially a hospitalization. This patient has a close social support with medical training, her mother, a registered nurse, who is staying with her during this crisis. If the mother does not feel she can manage the patient, and if there is no satisfactory safety plan in place, then she should be brought to the emergency room for further evaluation. If the mother is satisfied that she can manage the patient until her next

outpatient appointment, a trip to the emergency room might be avoided. Comorbid psychiatric illness may increase the likelihood of the patient attempting suicide or other self-injurious behaviors, so further evaluation during this urgent evening appointment suggests that a trip to the emergency room is warranted.

A2. _____ −2 The patient should be considered a safety risk as described in answer A1; however, she is not presently experiencing a panic attack, and a medium acting, fast-onset benzodiazepine such as alprazolam is not indicated.

A3. _____ −2 The patient's safety issues should be further investigated. There is no indication for the use of alprazolam as described in answer A2. CBT is one of the gold standard treatments for her anxiety and impulse-control issues; however, your evaluation of the patient is not complete enough to recommend a treatment course of strictly CBT. Establishing rapport with this patient is crucial, so sending her off to another specialist before determining the extent of her illness could possibly give her the impression that you are not aligned substantially. You also must educate the patient and her mother regarding your findings and the various treatments you may suggest once the evaluation is complete.

A4. _____ −2 It is true that the patient has a safety plan and there is no clear evidence that every patient who expresses passive suicidal ideation would benefit from hospitalization. Moreover, you have not completed your psychiatric evaluation, so you cannot know the extent of the illness, the presence of comorbid illnesses, or the psychosocial picture that would enable or hinder her ability to participate in treatment. These details could be drawn out in future sessions and the fact of establishing a therapeutic relationship with the patient may relieve some of her symptoms temporarily, enough to keep her out of the hospital and continue work with you. However, safety should be first on your mind. Additionally, you have no corroboration from her mother, with whom the patient says she would stay for safety. It is not yet clear whether this is a feasible plan.

A5. _____ +1 The key to this answer is that you have ruled out further evaluation in an emergency room for an ambivalently suicidal patient. The remainder of the answer is correct, regarding the additional information necessary for your evaluation with the addition of corroborative history from her mother, the person she asserts will keep her safe. You could evaluate this patient in your office and possibly arrange a satisfactory safety plan with the patient, but given the limited and worrisome information you have about the patient, she would probably benefit more from the safety and resources available in an emergency room.

DECISION POINT B

AXIS I:	(+2) Panic Disorder with Agoraphobia; (+2) Major Depressive Disorder, recurrent, without psychotic features; (+2) Obsessive-Compulsive Disorder; (−2) Social Phobia (Social Anxiety Disorder); (+2) Trichotillomania; (0) r/o Bipolar Disorder; (0) r/o Posttraumatic Stress Disorder; (−2) r/o Adjustment Disorder; Chronic; (−2) r/o Generalized Anxiety Disorder; r/o Anxiety Disorder, NOS
AXIS II:	(−2) r/o Obsessive-Compulsive Personality Disorder

Panic Disorder with Agoraphobia (+2). The patient accurately describes a panic attack, including palpitations, sweating, chest pain, dizziness, fear of dying, fear of losing control or going crazy, and nausea, having their apex within 10 minutes. For DSM-IV-TR diagnosis of a panic attack, a patient requires 4 of 13 symptoms. This patient endorses 6 and her account is corroborated by her mother. Other symptoms include trembling or shaking, sensations of shortness of breath or smothering, feeling of choking, derealization (feelings of unreality) or depersonalization (being detached from oneself), paresthesias (numbness or tingling sensations), and chills or hot flashes. She meets the criteria for agoraphobia because she is worried about having new attacks and subsequently stays home, which represents a significant change in behavior related to the attacks.

Major Depressive Disorder, Recurrent, Without Psychotic Features (+2). The patient describes feeling anhedonic and depressed, meeting both of criteria A for major depression when only one was required. She also has a diminished appetite, low energy, difficulty concentrating, and recurrent thoughts of death. These symptoms are not related to a medical illness and have contributed to an impairment in her social and academic/professional functioning. She does not currently abuse alcohol or substances, and these symptoms are not better accounted for by bereavement.

Obsessive-Compulsive Disorder (+2). This patient has a long history beginning in childhood of arranging her dolls in a certain order and repeating the process if she did not do it perfectly. She worried that if her food touched on her plate she would do something bad in school. She com-

plained that she had intrusive thoughts that made her anxious such as being a bad mother, requiring an "undoing" ritual of patting her head five times. She had to touch the right corner of a door jamb three times before entering a room or she would be sure someone in the room she was entering would hate her and she would have to leave. If she worried about someone hating her, she felt that the touching of the door jamb would protect her.

According to DSM-IV-TR:

A. Obsessions are defined by:
  1. recurrent and persistent thoughts, impulses, or images that are experienced, at some time during the disturbance, as intrusive and inappropriate and that cause marked anxiety or distress
  2. the thoughts, impulses, or images are not simply excessive worries about real-life problems
  3. the person attempts to ignore or suppress such thoughts, impulses, or images, or to neutralize them with some other thought or action
  4. the person recognizes that the obsessional thoughts, impulses, or images are the product of his or her own mind (not imposed from without as in thought insertion)

Compulsions are defined by:
  1. repetitive behaviors (e.g., hand washing, ordering, checking) or mental acts (e.g., praying, counting, repeating words silently) that the person feels driven to perform in response to an obsession, or according to rules that must be applied rigidly
  2. the behaviors or mental acts are aimed at preventing or reducing distress or preventing some dreaded

event or situation; however, these behaviors or mental acts either are not connected in a realistic way with what they are designed to neutralize or prevent or are clearly excessive

B. At some point during the course of the disorder, the person has recognized that the obsessions or compulsions are excessive or unreasonable. **Note:** This does not apply to children.

C. The obsessions or compulsions cause marked distress, are time consuming (take more than 1 hour a day), or significantly interfere with the person's normal routine, occupational (or academic) functioning, or usual social activities or relationships.

D. If another axis I disorder is present, the content of the obsessions or compulsions is not restricted to it (e.g., preoccupation with food in the presence of an Eating Disorder; hair pulling in the presence of Trichotillomania; concern with appearance in the presence of Body Dysmorphic Disorder; preoccupation with drugs in the presence of a Substance Use Disorder; preoccupation with having serious illness in the presence of Hypochondriasis; preoccupation with sexual urges or fantasies in the presence of a Paraphilia; or guilty ruminations in the presence of Major Depressive Disorder).

E. The disturbance is not due to the direct physiological effects of a substance (e.g., a drug of abuse, a medication) or a general medical condition.

Social Phobia (−2). Although this patient has described a marked and persistent fear of social situations, exposure to unfamiliar people or scrutiny by others, worrying that her behavior will be embarrassing or humiliating, she has developed compulsions to counteract the provoked anxiety. Her perceived negative scrutiny is also consistent with the agoraphobic feature of her panic disorder. Additionally, she describes intrusive thoughts that carry greater weight than a general worry about social situations, which until recently she was able to manage quite well, achieving high marks at very competitive academic institutions. She does not describe her panic attacks as provoked by a situation, but rather "out of the blue."

Trichotillomania (+2). You notice at her first visit that she is pulling her hair and there is hair loss behind her right ear. She admits she has been doing this for a while to relieve tension.

Rule Out Bipolar Disorder (0). The patient does not describe any symptoms consistent with this diagnosis except for some family history. Even though she does not present with bipolar disorder, you must obtain as much collateral information as possible to be sure she is not at risk for this disorder as the pharmacological treatment for OCD and major depressive disorder most certainly include SRIs, which could cause a mixed state. It seems highly unlikely in this patient, but you should carefully explore this possibility in your evaluation.

Rule Out Posttraumatic Stress Disorder (0). The patient was molested by her uncle for 2 years from 12–14 years of age. She does not provide a detailed description of this part of her life; however, there may be shared symptomatology with OCD, especially with her need to control aspects of her life. This molestation should be explored as a possible etiology for her symptoms given her history to help the therapist better understand the nature of her illness. However, at this stage there is little to support this diagnosis, such as the lack of nightmares, no restricted affect, no avoidance behaviors relating to, for example, her uncle or places where she might have been molested by her uncle.

Rule Out Adjustment Disorder, Chronic (−2). The patient does not describe a significant event or stressor that occurred within 6 months of the onset of symptoms. The stressor, if it is finding a job or moving back home to live with her mother, may be chronic, but her symptoms preceded this time frame.

Rule Out Generalized Anxiety Disorder (−2). This patient does describe excessive anxiety and worry about her future after completing her MBA, which is legitimate since she did not show up for interviews. She also describes having panic attacks in public and is having difficulty controlling the worry as evidenced by her OCD symptoms. She does not describe being restless or keyed up, easily fatigued, irritable, or having muscle tension. She only meets 2 of 6 criteria regarding the anxiety and worry, e.g., difficulty concentrating and sleep disturbance. She is worried about specific stressors rather than having general anxiety over numerous issues.

Rule Out Anxiety Disorder, Not Otherwise Specified (−2). Because this patient's symptoms can be better categorized as OCD and panic disorder with agoraphobia, this is not an appropriate diagnosis.

Rule Out Obsessive-Compulsive Personality Disorder (−2). There is evidence that the patient received comments about being inflexible and describes herself in terms that suggest some perfectionism and dedication to her work; however, she does not meet the criteria of a pervasive pattern of preoccupation with orderliness, perfectionism, and mental and interpersonal control, at the expense of flexibility, openness, and efficiency, beginning by early adulthood and present in a variety of contexts.

DECISION POINT C

C1. _____ +2 True
C2. _____ +2 False
C3. _____ +2 True
C4. _____ +2 False
C5. _____ +2 True
C6. _____ +2 False. The mean age at OCD onset ranges in epidemiological studies between 22 and 35 years, with at least one third of cases beginning by age 15 years.

C7. _____ +2 False. The heritability of panic disorder has been estimated to be approximately 43%.

C8. _____ +2 True

C9. _____ +2 True

C10. _____ +2 True

DECISION POINT D

D1. _____ +2 True. The therapeutic alliance is key to joining the therapist and the patient in a joint enterprise that will enable the patient to feel comfortable, especially while enduring therapeutic techniques such as ERP in which the patient must endure anxiety-provoking experiences for that anxiety to be relieved by desensitization. The therapist must gauge the aggressiveness of the treatment and the nuances of the patient's response to treatment and essentially understand the patient as much as possible to best facilitate a restructuring of his or her link between unwanted cognitions and behaviors.

D2. _____ −2 False. You can establish an educated diagnostic picture, but you would not avoid the process of building rapport as described in answer D1, nor would you send the patient off to another therapist or prescribe a medication to a medication-naive patient without first closely observing his or her response to treatment. This would be considered a dangerous action.

D3. _____ +2 True

D4. _____ +2 True

D5. _____ +2 True

D6. _____ +2 True

D7. _____ +2 True

D8. _____ +2 True

DECISION POINT E

E1. _____ +3 Starting with CBT and ERP alone is certainly acceptable. Given this patient's severity of symptoms plus major depressive symptoms, once you determine that she is not at risk for bipolar disorder and developing a mixed state from use of an SRI, you would probably want to begin treatment with pharmacotherapy simultaneously. Studies have shown that combination therapies of CBT with ERP and SRIs are more effective than CBT or medications alone. However, beginning with psychotherapy alone is still considered an effective strategy before starting medications. This patient has been through many medication trials and has never tried CBT with ERP, so she might prefer this approach. Starting with psychotherapy with this particular patient may be useful to build rapport and trust with you.

E2. _____ +5 Assuming you have ruled out bipolar disorder, this patient would benefit most from a more aggressive approach including both psychotherapy and psychopharmacotherapy. Studies have shown that combining therapies is more effective than monotherapy in some patients. Of course, you need to know what treatments she had with her prior psychiatrist so as not to repeat past failures

E3. _____ +3 Starting with an SRI alone is acceptable, especially if the patient has had good results in the past and does not wish to do psychotherapy. SRIs are the first-line treatment of choice because they have a better side effect profile than the older gold standard, clomipramine.

E4. _____ 0 Because of their relative safety compared with older medications such as clomipramine, the standard of care for treating OCD is to begin with SRIs. If the patient does not respond to the first trial of an SRI, studies suggest switching to a different SRI as it is difficult to determine an individual's response to each SRI. Clinical experience suggests that response rates to a second SRI trial are close to 50% but may diminish as the number of failed adequate trials increases. The initial treatment should be based upon the patient's medication history, and augmentation strategies are not appropriate as first-line treatment. Because we do not know the patient's history, and this question asks specifically for an initial treatment, considering augmentation to SRIs is not yet supported.

E5. _____ 0 If clomipramine is added, an augmentation strategy supported by at least three open-label studies, however, plasma concentration of clomipramine and desmethylclomipramine should be assayed 2–3 weeks after a dose of 50 mg/day is reached, and the total plasma concentration should be kept below 500 ng/ml to avoid cardiac and central nervous system toxicity. This answer assumes that the patient is already taking an SRI. Some clinicians might start the augmentation strategy if the initial SRI was not sufficiently effective. Others might choose a second SRI trial before beginning an augmentation strategy. This is an inappropriate option for an initial treatment because it implies that she is already taking a drug. As we do not know the patient's history, and this question asks specifically for an initial treatment, considering augmentation to SRIs is not yet supported.

SCORING

Decision Point	Score	Ideal Score
A		6
B		8
C		20
D		14
E		11
Total		59

KEY CLINICAL POINTS

1. The safest method for assessing suicidal ideation is face-to-face; comorbid psychiatric illness may increase the risk for a suicide attempt or self-injurious behavior.

2. In any psychotherapy, including intense anxiety-provoking exposure and response prevention (ERP), the strength of the therapeutic alliance is predictive of the patient's compliance and informs prognosis.

3. For obsessive-compulsive disorder, evidence indicates the most effective strategy for treatment includes both psychotherapy and psychopharmacotherapy.

REFERENCES

Abramowitz JS: Does cognitive-behavioral therapy cure obsessive-compulsive disorder? A meta-analytic evaluation of clinical significance. Behav Ther 1998; 29:355

American Psychiatric Association: Practice guideline for the treatment of patients with obsessive-compulsive disorder. Am J Psychiatry (in press)

Burke KC, Burke JD Jr., Regier DA, Rae DS: Age at onset of selected mental disorders in five community populations. Arch Gen Psychiatry 1990; 47:511–518

Cannon TD, Kaprio J, Lonnqvist J, Huttunen M, Koskenvuy M: The genetic epidemiology of schizophrenia in a Finnish twin cohort: a populationbased modeling study. Arch Gen Psychiatry 1998; 55:67–74

Carey G, Gottesman II: Twin and family studies of anxiety, phobic and obsessive disorders, in Anxiety: New Research and Changing Concepts. Edited by Klein DF, Rabkin J. New York, Raven Press, 1981, pp 117–136

Clifford CA, Murray RM, Fulker DW: Genetic and environmental influences on obsessional traits and symptoms. Psychol Med 1984; 14:791–800

Cottraux J, Bouvard MA, Milliery M: Combining pharmacotherapy with cognitive-behavioral interventions for obsessive-compulsive disorder. Cogn Behav Ther 2005; 34:185–192

Cottraux J, Note I, Yao SN, Lafont S, Note B, Mollard E, Bouvard M, Sauteraud A, Bourgeois M, Dartigues JF: A randomized controlled trial of cognitive therapy versus intensive behavior therapy in obsessive compulsive disorder. Psychother Psychosom 2001; 70:288–297

Eddy KT, Dutra L, Bradley R, Westen D: A multidimensional meta-analysis of psychotherapy and pharmacotherapy for obsessive-compulsive disorder. Clin Psychol Rev 2004; 24:1011–1030

Fisher PL, Wells A: How effective are cognitive and behavioral treatments for obsessive-compulsive disorder? A clinical significance analysis. Behav Res Ther 2005; 43:1543–1558

Freeston MH, Rheaume J, Ladouceur R: Correcting faulty appraisals of obsessional thoughts. Behav Res Ther 1996; 34:433–446

Goodman WK, Price LH, Rasmussen SA, Mzaure C, Fleischmann RL, Hill CL, Heninger GR, Charney DS: The Yale-Brown Obsessive Compulsive Scale. I. Development, use, and reliability. Arch Gen Psychiatry 1989; 46:1006–1011

Hettema JM, Neale MC, Kendler KS: A review and meta-analysis of the genetic epidemiology of anxiety disorders. Am J Psychiatry 2001; 158:1568–1578

Inouye E: Similar and dissimilar manifestations of obsessive-compulsive neuroses in monozygotic twins. Am J Psychiatry 1965; 121:1171–1175

Jonnal AH, Gardner CO, Prescott CA, Kendler KS: Obsessive and compulsive symptoms in a general population sample of female twins. Am J Med Genet 2000; 96:791–796

Ravizza L, Barzega G, Bellino S, Bogetto F, Maina G: Drug treatment of obsessive-compulsive disorder (OCD): long-term trial with clomipramine and selective serotonin reuptake inhibitors (SSRIs). Psychopharmacol Bull 1996; 32:167–173

Szegedi A, Wetzel H, Leal M, Hartter S, Hiemke C: Combination treatment with clomipramine and fluvoxamine: drug monitoring, safety, and tolerability data. J Clin Psychiatry 1996; 57:257–264

Van Balkom AJ, de Haan E, van Oppen P, Spinhoven P, Hoogduin KA, van Dyck R: Cognitive and behavioral therapies alone versus in combination with fluvoxamine in the treatment of obsessive compulsive disorder. J Nerv Ment Dis 1998; 186:492–499

Weissman MM, Bland RC, Canino GJ, Greenwald S, Hwu HG, Lee CK, Newman SC, Oakley-Browne MA, Rubio-Stipec M, Wickramaratne PJ, Wittchen H-U, Yeh E-K, the Cross National Collaborative Group: The cross national epidemiology of obsessive-compulsive disorder. J Clin Psychiatry 1994; 55(Mar suppl):5–10

Whittal ML, Thordarson DS, McLean PD: Treatment of obsessive-compulsive disorder: cognitive behavior therapy vs. exposure and response prevention. Behav Res Ther 2005; 43:1559–1576

7

Panic Disorder

I Can't Take Chances on My Heart

VIGNETTE PART 1

M is a 20-year-old male sophomore at an Ivy League College who presents to the school's teaching hospital emergency department (ED) with complaints of sharp chest pain, radiating down his left arm, numbness and tingling in his distal extremities, especially his hands and feet, heart palpitations, diaphoresis, and dizziness, all lasting approximately 5–7 minutes. The event had occurred approximately 45 minutes before his arrival to the hospital. He was driven to the ED by his college roommate. He continued to have a strong fear of dying and insisted that the staff "check my heart!" The ED resident quickly began a workup for myocardial infarction but soon discovered there were no diagnostic correlates on an electrocardiogram and laboratory studies to indicate that the patient had experienced a myocardial infarction. He consulted the on-call resident psychiatrist by phone and was instructed to draw blood for a complete blood count, comprehensive metabolic panel, and thyroid function tests and collect a urine sample for urinalysis and a urine toxicology screen. The patient's laboratory values were within normal limits except for positive screen results for cannabis. The psychiatrist asked the ED resident to give the patient lorazepam 1 mg i.v., given the intravenous line access from the earlier workup. Within 10 minutes the patient had calmed considerably and no longer feared his imminent death, but remained quite worried.

The on-call resident psychiatrist appeared within the next hour and began a psychiatric evaluation of the patient. M reported that he had never before experienced such an episode as the one that brought him to the ED. He appeared frightened, despite the treatment with lorazepam. He asked what happened, and the psychiatrist explained that it appeared he had a panic attack. He asked M what he was doing just before

the attack began. M reported that he was "hanging out with my roommate" and trying to motivate himself to study for an exam in 2 days' time. The roommate, still in the room, asked the psychiatrist how long the patient would be in the hospital because he had to get home and study. The psychiatrist told the roommate that the evaluation should not take much longer and they could leave together. He asked the roommate if he could please leave the room for privacy.

As the resident psychiatrist walked the roommate out of the patient's room to direct him to the waiting area, the roommate volunteered, "This test coming up is a big one. Physics. He needs to do well on it because he is pre-med." Then, he added, "I don't know if I'm off-base here, but he seems more—I don't know—depressed or worried or something. I know his girlfriend broke up with him a couple months ago—she's actually a good friend of mine—and she said she just couldn't take his moods anymore."

DECISION POINT A

Given what you know about this patient, was the decision by the resident psychiatrist to ask the ED resident to give the patient lorazepam 1 mg appropriate? Points awarded for correct and incorrect answers are scaled from best (5) to unhelpful but not harmful (0) to dangerous (−5).

A1. _____ The patient is suffering from severe anxiety due to the panic attack and administering a benzodiazepine intravenously is indicated to obtain near immediate relief of symptoms.

A2. _____ The patient is suffering from severe anxiety due to the panic attack and administering a benzodiazepine is indicated to obtain very quick relief of symptoms. However, giving it intravenously is not necessary.

A3. _____ The patient is suffering from severe anxiety due to the panic attack and administering a benzodiazepine is indicated to obtain very quick relief of symptoms. However, giving it intravenously is not a wise choice, given the patient's positive urine toxicology screen results for cannabis.

A4. _____ The patient has already calmed down and does not require benzodiazepine therapy.

A5. _____ The patient has already calmed down. You should start treatment with a selective serotonin reuptake inhibitor (SSRI) such as paroxetine or sertraline.

VIGNETTE PART 2

The patient tells the psychiatrist that he has been under a lot of pressure from his parents, especially his mother, to do well in school. He started school at a young age and turned 18 as a freshman in college. His birthday is at the end of December; instead of waiting a year to start kindergarten, he began early and has always been the youngest in his class. "You have to know my parents," he chuckled. He took a year off after his first year of college, uncertain about what he wanted to do and spending most of his time "partying, and being social, but not doing schoolwork." His parents expected him to become a doctor because his father is an orthopedic surgeon and his grandfather was a general practitioner. "I don't know if I want to become a doctor. *Definitely* not like my father. I don't think he understands people very well. My parents' friends are mostly my mother's. I've heard people are afraid to work with him. He got into trouble a couple of times for throwing scalpels! He has a horrible temper. But that is another story. He wouldn't agree, but I think he's an alcoholic. He and my mother both have two or three drinks every night. Martinis. They have a special setup in the dining room. Special glasses, the shaker, all of that. My mother is always threatening to divorce him. If I do become a doctor, I think I'll become something less stressful. I don't know. I guess it is not really my choice, though, since they're paying for it."

He is the oldest of three, with two younger sisters. "They're nothing like me. They don't have the pressure to become a doctor or a lawyer, although I think the older of the two is heading that way. She's just 2 years younger than me and she already volunteers at the public defender's office 1 day a week filing papers or something." The patient at first seemed relieved to talk about his history, but then suddenly announces, "Listen, man. I have to get back to my apartment. I have to study. Can I get more of that medication they gave me to calm down?"

The resident psychiatrist asks if there is any family history of mental illness, which the patient denies. He admits to smoking marijuana "occasionally, not like one of my roommates who is always stoned. I can't be stoned and do all this work." He then asks, "Do you think this is going to happen to me again? Or is it enough that I know about it? Will I be able to reason myself through it if I get nuts like this again?" He then continues, "I had a feeling it was in my head, but it is my heart, you know? I can't take chances on my heart." The resident psychiatrist agrees with his being careful and tells the patient it was wise to come to the emergency department. He then tells the patient he would like him to come back to the psychiatric outpatient department for a full evaluation to determine how to best help him. The patient agrees and is scheduled for an urgent appointment in 5 days.

DECISION POINT B

Given what you know about this patient, should you agree to his request and give him a supply of lorazepam to take home? What should you do? Points awarded for correct and incorrect answers are scaled from best (5) to unhelpful but not harmful (0) to dangerous (−5).

B1. _____ The patient has not offered you a specific stressor that causes the attacks suggesting that his attacks are unpredictable. For safety, you should give him five lorazepam 1 mg tablets to last him until his urgent appointment.

B2. _____ Despite not knowing the specific stressor, there probably is one. You simply have not had an opportunity to learn this yet. Individual therapy, to begin 5 days hence, will help elucidate the precipitant. Meanwhile, the patient requires protection from attacks with a benzodiazepine. Prescribe lorazepam 0.5 mg p.o. b.i.d. for now.

B3. _____ The patient has an urgent appointment in 5 days. Offer several nonpharmacological interventions he can perform himself should he again have a panic attack.

B4. _____ The patient demonstrated the use of cannabis, known for playing a role in potentiating panic attacks. Giving a known drug abuser lorazepam, a known drug of abuse, to take home is unwise because it is potentially dangerous if used inappropriately. Ask for permission to speak with the patient's family to gather additional medical and psychiatric history. In addition, if permission is obtained, ask the family to assist in monitoring the patient until his upcoming urgent appointment.

B5. _____ The patient has an urgent appointment in 5 days. Evaluate the patient for any additional psychiatric symptoms, which may require closer monitoring before his appointment.

VIGNETTE PART 3

You are now a psychiatrist working in the student mental health center of the patient's university. The patient arrives for his appointment 15 minutes late. He apologizes as he takes his seat and does not offer you eye contact. You ask how he is feeling today. He says, "I almost didn't come." There is a long pause. "I don't know," he tells you, "I just didn't want to leave my apartment. I haven't left it in the last 3 days. I'm missing classes, too." He appears somewhat disheveled, hair unkempt.

He is mildly malodorous. Once in his chair, he stares at his sneakers with his hair covering his eye. One of his thumbs taps the side of the chair quickly, then slowly, and then quickly again. You wait, noting that he is tearful.

"I'm—" he starts, "having a hard time. Really hard." He tells you that he has been feeling very depressed for several months now. "It's my parents. . . I don't know. . .my grades. . .my girlfriend. It's everything." He reports that his sleep has been disturbed for at least a year, with difficulty initiating sleep and frequent awakenings. He typically ruminates about the issues bothering him until he finally falls asleep; then often he has been sleeping late, sometimes until noon or 1:00 p.m., subsequently missing classes. His grades have been deteriorating over the course of the year, at first gradually, but in the last 2 months he has stopped attending many of his classes and is in danger of finishing the term on academic probation.

Decision Point C

Which of the following statements regarding the epidemiology of panic disorder and comorbid psychiatric diagnoses are true and which are false? (2) points awarded for answering correctly.

T F C1. _____ Panic disorder has a lifetime prevalence of approximately 1.6%–2.2%

T F C2. _____ Panic disorder may present first in prepubescent children, although this is relatively uncommon.

T F C3. _____ When panic disorder presents in adolescence, it occurs more frequently in boys than in girls, by a factor of 2:1.

T F C4. _____ Panic disorder is classified in the DSM-IV-TR as having two subtypes: with agoraphobia and without agoraphobia. The lifetime prevalence of the subtype with agoraphobia is approximately 20%.

T F C5. _____ Approximately one third of patients with panic disorder are depressed when they present for treatment.

T F C6. _____ Patients with panic disorder who have co-occurring depression have a lower risk for suicide attempts.

T F C7. _____ Patients with panic disorder are less likely to seek treatment than those with other psychiatric disorders.

T F C8. _____ Panic disorder has been shown to have a very strong familial pattern of inheritance.

T F C9. _____ Abuse of substances and alcohol is very high among patients with panic disorder, irrespective of subtype.

T F C10. _____ Between 40 and 50% of patients with panic disorder also meet criteria for one or more axis II disorders strictly from cluster B (antisocial personality disorder, histrionic personality disorder, borderline personality disorder, and narcissistic personality disorder).

Decision Point D

Match the following types of psychotherapy with their corresponding descriptions (2) points awarded for correct answer.

Type of Therapy	Description
___D1. Cognitive behavioral therapy	A. Based on the theory that unrecognized emotions (typically triggered by interpersonal situations) trigger panic attacks; therefore, patients are encouraged in a methodical manner, emphasized with exercises and homework, to explore and process their emotional reactions with the aim of reducing or eliminating anxieties surrounding these targeted emotions.
___D2. Supportive psychotherapy	B. Decreases shame and stigma, offers opportunities for modeling, inspiration, and reinforcement, provides a naturally occurring exposure environment especially good for patients experiencing fear of panic symptoms in social situations.
___D3. Group therapy	C. Based on the assumption that maladaptive patterns of cognition and behavior maintain panic disorder.
___D4. Eye-movement desensitization and reprocessing	D. 12-week manualized treatment program, delivered twice weekly, that focuses on the underlying psychological meaning of panic symptoms and on current social and emotional functioning.
___D5. Panic focused psychodynamic psychotherapy	E. Eight-stage process during which the patient attends to past and present experiences in brief sequential doses while simultaneously focusing on an external stimulus. The process is repeated with the intention of focusing this dual attention and personal association in a more adaptive fashion.

ANSWERS: SCORING, RELATIVE WEIGHTS, AND COMMENTS

DECISION POINT A

A1. _____ −5 There is no indication for administering intravenous benzodiazepine medications to a patient whose symptoms have abated. Although benzodiazepines for panic disorder have been demonstrated to be useful for patients whose symptoms are particularly distressing and impairing and for whom rapid control is critical, giving benzodiazepines to patients with presumed substance abuse (tested positive for cannabis) should be avoided whenever possible. These patients have a higher prevalence of benzodiazepine abuse, a greater euphoric response to benzodiazepines, and a higher rate of unauthorized use of alprazolam during treatment.

A2. _____ −5 For the same reasons stated in answer A1, giving benzodiazepines to a patient with a presumed substance abuse problem is not advised. Moreover, the patient's symptoms have abated enough that the wiser choice of treatment would be connecting the patient to a psychiatrist and/or psychotherapist who could follow the patient and offer more effective long-term treatments such as cognitive behavior therapy with or without psychopharmacological agents such as an SSRI.

A3. _____ −3 Although this answer addresses the issue of the patient's positive toxicology screen results for cannabis, suggesting abuse, and further suggesting the preference for alternative treatments, it does not account for the abatement of the acute symptoms and subsequently for an opportunity to choose a more effective long-term treatment strategy such as cognitive behavior therapy with or without psychopharmacological agents such as an SSRI.

A4. _____ +5 This answer is true. It does not offer other possible treatment options, but the question does not require this.

A5. _____ −3 Although treatment of panic disorder with SSRIs such as sertraline or paroxetine is certainly indicated, you are an ED psychiatrist and unless you continue to see this patient as an outpatient, prescribing long-term psychopharmacological treatments is not considered safe practice.

DECISION POINT B

B1. _____ −5 There is the possibility the patient has a substance abuse problem given his positive toxicology screen results for cannabis. Giving even a small amount of benzodiazepines to take home is not safe practice. Moreover, despite his negative toxicology screen results for benzodiazepines, he may still abuse them, as the threshold for positive results does not necessarily account for low-dose prescriptions. High-dose abuse of benzodiazepines can result in positive urine toxicology screen results for up to 6–8 weeks after the last use.

B2. _____ −5 If the patient had not demonstrated a positive toxicology screen for cannabis, this would be an acceptable treatment plan.

B3. _____ +3 This is a wise plan. Deep breathing exercises, rebreathing of CO_2 in a paper bag, guided imagery, finding a supportive friend or relative to help calm the patient during the attack, and other techniques are likely to help in the short-run, before the patient engages in more substantive therapy. An emphasis on finding a supportive environment should be stressed, however. The prevalence of comorbid axis I or axis II diagnoses increases the patient's risk for suicide, even though the literature on suicidality or attempts in the context of panic disorder as the single diagnosis is still considered controversial.

B4. _____ +5 This is a sound, rational plan.

B5. _____ +5 There is a high prevalence of comorbid axis I or axis II diagnoses concurrent with panic disorder. It is essential to explore the patient's symptoms and history for more information to help guide immediate treatment options.

DECISION POINT C

C1. _____ T Weissman et al. collected epidemiologic data from multiple countries and noted a similar lifetime prevalence of approximately 1.6%–2.2%.

C2. _____ T Panic disorder may have an onset before puberty, although this is less common.

C3. _____ F There is a higher risk for panic disorder in females during adolescence (approximately 2:1). The lifetime prevalence is also approximately twice as high in women than in men. Moreover, women are more likely to have panic disorder with agoraphobia than men.

C4. _____ T There are two subtypes as described; the prevalence of the agoraphobic subtype is approximately 20%.

C5. _____ T The lifetime prevalence of major depression as a comorbid diagnosis with panic disorder without agoraphobia is approximately 34.7% and is 38.7% for panic disorder with agoraphobia. The onset of depression has been found to occur with or after the onset of panic disorder in approximately two-thirds of patients and precede the onset of panic disorder in one-third.

C6. _____ F Given the high comorbidity of panic disorders with mood disorders as stated in answer C5, plus the associated risk of suicidal ideation, attempts, and completion with mood disorders uncomplicated by panic disorder, the risk of suicide with complicated panic disorder is higher. In addition, these patients have a higher risk for impaired social and marital functioning, work impairment, use of psychoactive medication, and substance abuse.

C7. _____ F Patients with panic disorder are more likely than those with other psychiatric disorders to seek treatment relatively frequently. They more often seek help from nonpsychiatrists and from EDs.

C8. _____ T The results of multinational studies have shown a median risk of panic disorder to be eight times as high in the first-degree relatives of probands with panic disorder as in the relatives of control subjects. Early-onset panic disorder demonstrated the greatest familial risk, at approximately 17 times greater.

C9. _____ T Irrespective of panic disorder subtype, clinical and epidemiological studies have demonstrated a higher than average rate of substance and alcohol abuse and dependence. Interestingly, approximately 50% of those with panic disorder had prior onset of the comorbid substance or alcohol abuse/dependence disorder.

C10. _____ F It is true that 40%–50% of patients with panic disorder will also meet criteria for one or more of the axis II disorders; however, they typically have been shown to have many of the traits associated with cluster B personalities, such as affective instability from borderline personality disorder, impulsivity from borderline personality disorder or antisocial personality disorder, and hypersensitivity to people from paranoid personality disorder. The most common personality disorders most frequently diagnosed fall in cluster C, sometimes known as the "anxious" cluster: avoidant personality disorder, obsessive-compulsive personality disorder, and dependent personality disorder. At least one study of longitudinal data has suggested that the early onset of panic disorder predicts a subsequent onset of personality disorders.

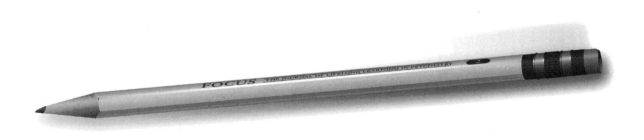

DECISION POINT D

Type of Therapy	Description
D1._____ C. Cognitive behavioral therapy. Based on the assumption that maladaptive patterns of cognition and behavior maintain panic disorder.	Probably the most extensively studied nonpharmacological intervention; cognitive behavior therapy (CBT) has been shown to be effective in treating the targeted symptoms of panic disorder and also helps to reduce the frequency and severity of co-occurring conditions. It is the most commonly used psychotherapy for panic and other anxiety disorders. Panic-focused in a circumscribed course of 10–15 weekly sessions. There is growing evidence, partly conflicting, that concurrent use of medications (such as imipramine, fluvoxamine, or benzodiazepines) with CBT may either work synergistically in the acute phase or actually hinder the long-term effects of the CBT. More studies are needed.
D2._____ A. Supportive psychotherapy. Based on the theory that unrecognized emotions (typically triggered by interpersonal situations) trigger panic attacks; therefore, patients are encouraged in a methodical manner, emphasized with exercises and homework, to explore and process their emotional reactions with the aim of reducing or eliminating anxieties surrounding these targeted emotions.	Considered less effective than CBT or medications in the treatment of panic disorder. The effect in studies was similar to that of placebo. Thus, this type of psychotherapy is not recommended for the treatment of panic disorder.
D3._____ B. Group therapy. Decreases shame and stigma, offers opportunities for modeling, inspiration, and reinforcement, provides a naturally occurring exposure environment especially good for patients experiencing fear of panic symptoms in social situations.	Only group CBT therapy has been demonstrated as being effective in controlled studies. Evidence on the effectiveness of other approaches, such as mindfulness-based stress reduction, in group settings is limited. Other untested group approaches, such as medication support groups, may be effective as adjunctive treatments.
D4._____ E. Eye-movement desensitation and reprocessing. Eight-stage process during which the patient attends to past and present experiences in brief sequential doses while simultaneously focusing on an external stimulus. The process is repeated with the intention of focusing this dual attention and personal association in a more adaptive fashion.	Developed primarily for posttraumatic stress disorder, this modality has been studied more recently for the treatment of panic disorder. There have not been substantial studies, however, and one study found the effects of this method to be equivalent to those of placebo. Thus, this type of treatment was not recommended for the treatment of panic disorder.
D5._____ D. Panic focused psychodynamic psychotherapy. 12-week manualized treatment program, delivered twice weekly, that focuses on the underlying psychological meaning of panic symptoms and on current social and emotional functioning.	Developed by Milrod, this 12-week manualized treatment based on basic assumptions of insight-oriented psychodynamic psychotherapy, but unlike other psychodynamic-oriented approaches, is narrower in focus. Patients must confront the underlying assumption that their panic symptoms are motivated by difficulty separating from important attachment figures and perceiving themselves as autonomous. This theory suggests that patients with panic disorder develop an agoraphobic avoidance, triggered by high levels of anxiety, as they perceive their environment and relationships as dangerous coupled with an inadequacy and lack of autonomy within themselves. Panic focused psychodynamic psychotherapy has been tested in a randomized control study, but its greatest efficacy has been shown when it is used adjunctively with CBT and pharmacotherapy.

YOUR TOTAL

Decision Point	Score	Ideal Score
A		5
B		13
C		20
D		10
Total		48

KEY CLINICAL POINTS

1. Unless follow-up is assured for a patient presenting in the emergency room, the psychiatrist should not prescribe medications.

2. Knowledge of epidemiology and potential comorbidities may assist the psychiatrist in understanding the patient. Panic disorder has a lifetime prevalence of approximately 1.6%–2.2%, it is less likely to have an onset before puberty, there is an approximate 2:1 ratio of females to males during adolescence, and the lifetime prevalence of comorbid major depression with panic disorder is approximately 34.7% to 38.7%.

3. The most extensively studied psychotherapeutic intervention for panic disorder is cognitive behavioral therapy (CBT).

REFERENCES

Alonso J, Angermeyer MC, Bernert S, Bruffaerts R, Brugha TS, Bryson H, de Girolamo G, Graaf R, Demyttenaere K, Gasquet I, Haro JM, Katz SJ, Kessler RC, Kovess V, Lépine JP, Ormel J, Polidori G, Russo LJ, Vilagut G, Almansa J, Arbabzadeh-Bouchez S, Autonell J, Bernal M, Buist-Bouwman MA, Codony M, Domingo-Salvany A, Ferrer M, Joo SS, Martínez-Alonso M, Matschinger H, Mazzi F, Morgan Z, Morosini P, Palacín C, Romera B, Taub N, Vollebergh WA, ESEMeD/MHEDEA 2000 Investigators, European Study of the Epidemiology of Mental Disorders (ESEMeD) Project: Disability and quality of life impact of mental disorders in Europe: results from the European Study of the Epidemiology of Mental Disorders (ESEMeD) project. Acta Psychiatr Scand Suppl 2004; 38–46

Barlow DH, Craske MG, Cerney JA, Klosko JS: 1. Behavioral treatment of panic disorder. Behav Ther 1989; 20:261–282

Boyd JH: Use of mental health services for the treatment of panic disorder. Am J Psychiatry 1986; 143:1569–1574

Brown TA, Barlow DH: Long-term outcome in cognitive-behavioral treatment of panic disorder: clinical predictors and alternative strategies for assessment. J Consult Clin Psychol 1995; 63:754–765

Busch FN, Shapiro T: The panic patient, Psychodynamic Concepts in General Psychiatry. Edited by Schwartz HJ, Bleiberg E, Weissman SH. Washington, DC, American Psychiatric Press, 1995, pp 249–262

Cameron OG, Hill EM: Women and anxiety. Psychiatr Clin North Am 1989; 12:175–186

Cerny JA, Barlow DH, Craske MG, Himadi WG: Couples treatment of agoraphobia: a 20 two-year follow-up. Behav Ther 1987; 18:401–415

Ciraulo DA, Sands BF, Shader RI: Critical review of liability for benzodiazepine abuse among alcoholics. Am J Psychiatry 1988; 145:1501–1506

den Boer JA, Westenberg HG: Effect of a serotonin and noradrenaline uptake inhibitor in panic disorder; a double-blind comparative study with fluvoxamine and maprotiline. Int Clin Psychopharmacol 1988; 3:59–74

Eaton WW, Dryman A, Weissman MM: Panic and phobia, in Psychiatric Disorders in America. Edited by Robins LN, Regier DA. New York, Free Press, 1991, pp 155–179

Fleet RP, Marchand A, Dupuis G, Kaczorowski J, Beitman BD: Comparing emergency department and psychiatric setting patients with panic disorder. Psychosomatics 1998; 39:512–518

Gabbard GO: Panic disorder, in Psychodynamic Psychiatry in Clinical Practice, 4th ed. Washington, DC, American Psychiatric Press, 2002, pp 253–259

Goodwin RD, Brook JS, Cohen P: Panic attacks and the risk of personality disorder. Psychol Med 2005; 35:227–235

Goodwin RD, Hamilton SP: Lifetime comorbidity of antisocial personality disorder and anxiety disorders among adults in the community. Psychiatry Res 2003; 117: 159–166

Goldstein RB, Wickramaratne PJ, Horwath E, Weissman MM: Familial aggregation and phenomenology of "early'-onset (at or before age 20 years) panic disorder. Arch Gen Psychiatry 1997; 54:271–278

Hoffart A, Thornes K, Hedley LM: DSM-III-R axis I and II disorders in agoraphobic inpatients with and without panic disorder before and after psychosocial treatment. Psychiatry Res 1995; 56:1–9

Jacobi F, Wittchen HU, Holting C, Hofler M, Pfister H, Müller N, Lieb R: Prevalence, comorbidity and correlates of mental disorders in the general population: results from the German Health Interview and Examination Survey (GHS). Psychol Med, 2004; 34:597–611

Kabat-Zinn J, Massion AO, Kristeller J, Peterson LG, Fletcher KE, Pbert L, Lenderking WR, Santorelli SF: Effectiveness of a meditation-based stress reduction program in the treatment of anxiety disorders. Am J Psychiatry 1992; 149:936–943

Kessler RC, Chiu WT, Jin R, Ruscio AM, Shear K, Walters EE: The epidemiology of panic attacks, panic disorder, and agoraphobia in the National Comorbidity Survey Replication. Arch Gen Psychiatry 2006; 63:415–424

Klerman GL, Weissman MM, Ouellette R, Johnson J, Greenwald S: Panic attacks in the community. Social morbidity and health care utilization. JAMA 1991; 265:742–746

Knowles JA, Weissman MM: Panic disorder and agoraphobia, in American Psychiatric Press Review of Psychiatry. Edited by Oldham JM, Riba MB. Washington, DC, American Psychiatric Press, 1995, pp 383–404

Lidren DM, Watkins PL, Gould RA, Clum GA, Asterino M, Tulloch HL: A comparison of bibliotherapy and group therapy in the treatment of panic disorder. J Consult Clin Psychol 1994; 62:865–869

Markowitz JS, Weissman MM, Ouellette R, Lish JD, Klerman GL: Quality of life in panic disorder. Arch Gen Psychiatry 1989; 46:984–992

Mavissakalian M: The relationship between panic disorder/agoraphobia and personality disorders. Psychiatr Clin North Am 1990; 13:661–684

Miller JJ, Fletcher K, Kabat-Zinn J: Three-year follow-up and clinical implications of a mindfulness meditation-based stress reduction intervention in the treatment of anxiety disorders. Gen Hosp Psychiatry 1995; 17:192–200

Milrod B, Busch F, Cooper A, Shapiro T: Manual of Panic-Focused Psychodynamic Psychotherapy. Washington, DC, American Psychiatric Press, 1997

Milrod B, Busch F, Leon AC, Aronson A, Roiphe J, Rudden M, Rudden M, Singer M, Goldman H, Richter D, Shear MK: A pilot open trial of brief psychodynamic psychotherapy for panic disorder. J Psychother Pract Res, 2001; 10:239–245

Milrod B, Busch F, Leon AC, Shapiro T, Aronson A, Roiphe J, Rudden M, Singer M, Goldman H, Richter D, Shear MK: Open trial of psychodynamic psychotherapy for panic disorder: a pilot study. Am J Psychiatry 2000; 157:1878–1880

Neron S, Lacroix D, Chaput Y: Group vs individual cognitive behaviour therapy in panic disorder: an open clinical trial with a six month follow-up. Can J Behav Sci 1995; 27:379–392

Reich J, Noyes R Jr, Troughton E: Dependent personality disorder associated with phobic avoidance in patients with panic disorder. Am J Psychiatry 1987; 144: 323–326

Sareen J, Cox BJ, Afifi TO, de Graaf R, Asmundson GJ, ten Have M, Stein MB: Anxiety disorders and risk for suicidal ideation and suicide attempts: a population-based longitudinal study of adults. Arch Gen Psychiatry 2005; 62:1249–1257

Sareen J, Stein MB, Cox BJ, Hassard ST: Understanding comorbidity of anxiety disorders with antisocial behavior: findings from two large community surveys. J Nerv Ment Dis 2004; 192:178–186

Schatzberg AF, Nemeroff CB: The American Psychiatric Publishing Textbook of Psychopharmacology, 3rd ed. Washington, DC, American Psychiatric Publishing, 2004

Shear MK, Houck P, Greeno C, Masters S: Emotion-focused psychotherapy for patients with panic disorder. Am J Psychiatry 2001; 158:1993–1998

Shelton RC, Harvey DS, Stewart PM, Loosen PT: Alprazolam in panic disorder: a retrospective analysis. Prog Neuropsychopharmacol Biol Psychiatry 1993; 17: 423–434

Telch MJ, Lucas JA, Schmidt NB, Hanna HH, LaNae JT, Lucas RA: Group cognitive-behavioral treatment of panic disorder. Behav Res Ther 1993; 31:279–287

Thyer BA, Himle J, Curtis GC, Cameron OG, Nesse RM: A comparison of panic disorder and agoraphobia with panic attacks. Compr Psychiatry 1985; 26:208–214

Tsao JC, Lewin MR, Craske MG: The effects of cognitive-behavior therapy for panic disorder on comorbid conditions. J Anxiety Disord 1998; 12:357– 371

Tsao JCI, Mystkowski J, Zucker B, Craske MG: Effects of cognitive behavioral therapy for panic disorder on comorbid conditions: replication and extension. Behav Ther 2002; 33:493–509

Tsao JC, Mystkowski JL, Zucker BG, Craske MG: Impact of cognitive-behavioral therapy for panic disorder on comorbidity: a controlled investigation. Behav Res Ther 2005; 43:959–970

Wang PS, Lane M, Olfson M, Pincus HA, Wells KB, Kessler RC: Twelve-month use of mental health services in the United States: results from the National Comorbidity Survey Replication. Arch Gen Psychiatry 2005; 62: 629–640

Watanabe N, Churchill R, Furukawa TA (2007). Combination of psychotherapy and benzodiazepines versus either therapy alone for panic disorder: a systematic review. BMC Psychiatry 2007; 7:18

Weissman MM, Bland RC, Canino GJ, Faravelli C, Greenwald S, Hwu HG, Joyce PR, Karam EG, Lee CK, Lellouch J, Lépine JP, Newman SC, Oakley-Browne MA, Rubio-Stipec M, Wells JE, Wickramaratne PJ, Wittchen HU, Yeh EK: The cross-national epidemiology of panic disorder. Arch Gen Psychiatry 1997; 54:305–309

Weissman MM, Klerman GL, Markowitz JS, Ouellette R: Suicidal ideation and suicide attempts in panic disorder and attacks. N Engl J Med 1989; 321:1209–1214

8

Personality Disorders

The Construction of a Young Woman

VIGNETTE

You are a psychiatrist in private practice. Susan, a 28-year-old divorced woman, was referred after release from an inpatient psychiatric unit at a local hospital. She was admitted 3 weeks prior for worsening symptoms of depression and a suicide attempt, in which she overdosed on a total of 3 grams of acetaminophen, 20 mg of alprazolam, 4000 mg of valproic acid, and 10 mg of risperidone. After a brief stay on the general medical ward, she was transferred to the inpatient psychiatric unit for further observation and stabilization of her mood. This was her fourth suicide attempt in the past year, and it was her sixth psychiatric hospitalization, four of which had occurred in the past 2 years. You agreed to see her as part of the patient's discharge disposition because the referral came from a colleague who felt you would be best suited to treat her given your experience with patients whose primary diagnosis falls under axis II.

You receive a copy of her admission note and discharge summary. You learn that the patient was born to a New York City family and was the oldest of three children, with one brother and one sister. She alleged physical, sexual, and emotional abuse by her father, her uncle, and her father's friend beginning at age 6 and continuing for 3 years. She was taken from her family by child protective services and placed in foster care for 9 months, then reunited after the father moved away. No charges were brought against him, but her mother often told her, "This is all your fault. He only tried to help you." When questioned further about her experiences, she responded, tearfully, "I can't talk about them. I'm sorry. I just put that stuff away and there it will stay. People just want to hurt me. I've never known love."

She attended private school and did well in her classes until her junior year, when her grades began to dip. She

started using alcohol to excess on weekends, drinking to the point of passing out, and by the time she was a senior she was also smoking marijuana and using Ecstasy. She made her first suicide attempt that year by superficially cutting her wrists. The injuries did not require hospitalization, but her family sent her to a private inpatient substance abuse rehabilitation center; she spent 30 days there, became sober, and began to attend Alcoholics Anonymous meetings. She relapsed approximately 2 months later, then spent another week in an intensive outpatient rehabilitation program. After that, she remained sober through college. Her cutting became habitual, and she continued to cut her thighs periodically with an antique pocket knife her uncle had given her that she kept in her purse—the same uncle who allegedly sexually abused her. She could go for several months at a time without cutting, but certain triggers, sometimes real, sometimes imagined, would cause her to return to this self-mutilating behavior. She admitted to cutting for approximately 2 weeks prior to her most recent admission.

She had a series of casual sexual relationships during her years at a small New England college, some with men and some with women. She maintained a long-term relationship with her boyfriend, who attended an Ivy League school 100 miles away, and did not tell him about her affairs. Her relationships with her peers were rocky, and she developed a reputation for being "moody," often turning on her friends for alleged slights. On two occasions her friends reported to her that she had disappeared from her dormitory room and returned 2 or 3 days later, disheveled, tired, wearing the same clothes, but unclear where she had been. Her friends assumed that she had been "partying hard" on Ecstasy, and no one pursued the incidents any further.

Her mood continued to deteriorate during college. Despite maintaining high grades, she had increasing thoughts of suicide and made at least two more attempts by overdosing on medications she took from friends. None of these attempts required hospitalization. Eventually one of her friends convinced her to seek psychiatric help, and she began seeing a therapist weekly and a psychiatrist every 6 weeks for medical management. She was started on citalopram, but after 1 week she complained of stomach pain and jitteriness and was switched to venlafaxine. This drug seemed to help her for approximately 3 months, when she was switched to bupropion because of sexual side effects. During the next 2 years she reports having been on valproic acid, lithium, carbamazepine, risperidone, fluoxetine, paroxetine, buspirone, clonazepam, lorazepam, and temazepam. Currently she takes 60 mg of duloxetine daily, 40 mg of aripiprazole twice daily, and 150 mg of trazodone at bedtime. Her therapies mostly consisted of psychodynamic psychotherapy and cognitive behavior therapy, with which she experienced marginal improvement of symptoms. Her last psychiatrist was convinced that she had bipolar I disorder, but she quit seeing him when he refused to prescribe alprazolam for her.

The patient shows up to her scheduled appointment 10 minutes late, and before she can remove her stylish leather coat, she explains that it is not her fault that she is not on time, but her current boyfriend "simply refused to realize how important these appointments are." Her coat is appropriate for the fall weather, but her black skirt rides quite high on her thighs. She is wearing a low-cut blouse, and her hair has magenta highlights. She sits down opposite you, crosses her legs, and says, "I know the deal. I tell you all about my history of sexual, emotional, and physical abuse by my father, my uncle, and my father's best friend— oh, and my brother, too—and how many times I've tried to kill myself. I actually love my uncle despite all of that. He was the nicest one in my family. He is an architect, so I know he's smart. You ask me what meds I'm on, if I'm still suicidal, and then we change the meds."

She says her current medications have been working for the past 6 months, but she heard there is a new sleeping pill, eszopiclone, and she would like to try it. Before you have a chance to say anything, she continues: "I graduated magna cum laude with a degree in psychology, so I know a lot. You can talk to me like an equal." Her story continues with a brief history of her work experience as a copy editor for a well-known fashion magazine in New York City, which she quit after 6 months because, she says, "the boss kept grabbing my ass and it was bringing back bad memories. She was convinced I was a dyke, but I'm not completely dyke. Just some of the time. I'd say I'm a dyke during the week and totally heterosexual on the weekends. Do you think that's strange? Anyway, that boss was an idiot, and I didn't want to work there anyway."

She tells you she felt lonely and had no friends she could trust in New York, despite having family who live there. "Most people just don't get me. They think I'm full of shit or they have their pretty lives and they have no idea what it is to struggle. I can't stand most people. They really irritate me. I often start screaming at them for no reason. I know that freaks them out, but so what. They don't understand me. Some of them, my girlfriends in college, tried to help me, but I didn't let them." Her last relationship was a marriage that ended in divorce after 3 years because her husband, the same longterm boyfriend from her early college days, was unfaithful and she "could not be married to someone I can't trust." Before the marriage, they had gone through a series of breakups and reconciliations from the time she was a senior in high school. "We should not have gotten married," she says, "especially after being together for so long. We used to fight all the time because he was jealous. He hated when I spoke to anyone, even girls. But he knew I could go either way, so I guess he had a reason to be jealous." She laughs. "Of course, I did cheat on him all the time. But I had to. I'm a girl! He would not come visit me. He was an asshole from the first day I met him. I used to think he was my dream man until I got to know him. Then it was a matter of how to get rid of him." You notice she punctuates a lot of her sentences with exaggerated sighs, snorts, and chortles. "He was also jealous that I was smarter than him. I tried never to make him feel insecure. God, that would be the last thing I would do. I like to help people. I don't want them to be intimidated by me." Then she becomes tearful. "I was abused," she sobs. "I'll never get over it. I don't care if you make me comatose."

She admits to drinking at least three or four times during the week, sometimes by herself "to help me sleep. These drugs just don't do it." She has tried to cut down on her drinking—"because I think it's going to make me fat at some point, at least if I start eating as well"—and on her use of other drugs. "I like Ecstasy, I have to admit. It makes you feel loved by everybody. I don't have that in my life without E. But I know it's not good to keep doing that. I started with just one tab, but now I need at least six to get going. I usually keep two more for later. But I know someone whose brain turned to mush." She admits to having had sexual relations in the past with two different men who were drug dealers in order to obtain drugs when she was low on cash. "I'll never do that again," she says. "They were both just mean jerks about it. I mean, I was willing to give them a little, you know, but they were violent. They liked to hold me down and make me scream for them. I had bruises."

DECISION POINT A

Given this presentation, what is your differential diagnosis for axis I and axis II, according to the DSM-IV-TR criteria?

AXIS I:	
AXIS II:	

DECISION POINT B

Given the information presented, how would you assess her suicide risk? What steps should you take? (There may be more than one correct answer. Mark as many as you believe are correct. Points are deducted for incorrect answers.)

B1. _____ Definite. The patient has made several attempts in the past and was just hospitalized for a suicide attempt, and you know that 8%–10% of borderline patients successfully commit suicide. You should create a contract for safety and develop a clear safety plan with this patient immediately.

B2. _____ Likely. The patient has made several attempts in the past. She has not made any since her last discharge, and she showed up (albeit late) at her appointment to see you. This is a good sign that she is trying to help herself and is not engaged in self-destructive behavior. However, her last attempt was so recent that she cannot be fully trusted. Create a contract for safety with the patient and develop a clear safety plan immediately.

B3. _____ Impossible to say. There are no guaranteed methods for assessing the likelihood of a person's committing suicide. We only have statistical evidence that suggests that this patient is in a high-risk category. This does not mean that she will or will not commit suicide.

B4. _____ Impossible to say. You need to assess her suicide risk by asking pertinent questions about her feelings of rejection, her fear of abandonment, and how she is managing the transition from the structured environment of the hospital to living on her own.

B5. _____ Impossible to say. Assess her suicide risk as suggested in B4, but consider that she has some comorbid disorders that increase the likelihood that she will make another attempt in the immediate future. You can manage her as an outpatient, and if she begins to demonstrate deterioration of mood and increased suicidal ideation, send her to the closest emergency room for safety. Meanwhile, arrange for her to begin a dialectical behavior therapy group and/or individual therapy at your outpatient clinic. Additionally, the patient requires substance use treatment, which is categorically imperative to any success in other therapies.

DECISION POINT C

According to current evidence supported by two or more randomized, placebo-controlled, doubleblind trials, what are the most effective psychopharmacological treatment recommendations for affective dysregulation symptoms, impulse-behavioral dyscontrol symptoms, and cognitive-perceptual symptoms in patients with borderline personality disorder? For each class, fill in the appropriate drugs if they meet the above mentioned evidence-based criteria. (One point is given for each correctly placed drug. Two points are deducted for incorrect answers.)

Drug Class	Affective Dysregulation Symptoms[a]	Impulse-Behavioral Dyscontrol Symptoms[b]	Cognitive-Perceptual Symptoms[c]
SSRIs and related antidepressants			
MAOIs			
Mood stabilizers			
Benzodiazepines			
Atypical antipsychotics			
Conventional antipsychotics			

SSRIs = selective serotonin reuptake inhibitors; MAOIs = monoamine oxidase inhibitors
[a]Affective dysregulation symptoms include depressed mood, mood lability, rejection sensitivity, anxiety, impulsivity, self-mutilation, anger/hostility, psychoticism, poor global functioning, and behavioral dyscontrol.
[b]Impulse-behavioral dyscontrol symptoms include impulsive aggression, anger, irritability, self-injurious behavior, and poor global functioning.
[c]Cognitive-perceptual symptoms include ideas of reference, illusions, paranoid ideation, and associated anger/hostility.

DECISION POINT D

Given the patient's presentation and DSM-IV-TR criteria, could you make the diagnosis of posttraumatic stress disorder (PTSD)?

D1. _____ Yes. The patient suffered multiple sexual assaults as a young woman.

D2. _____ No. Sexual assault by itself is not enough to make the diagnosis.

DECISION POINT E

What is the epidemiology of borderline personality disorder? For each statement, answer "true" or "false." (Two points are given for correct answers, and 2 points are deducted for incorrect answers.)

E1. _____ It is the second most common personality disorder in clinical settings, after narcissistic and histrionic personality disorders, which are tied for first at 15% each.

E2. _____ It is the most common personality disorder in clinical settings, present in 20% of all psychiatric outpatients and 30%–35% of psychiatric inpatients.

E3. _____ It is the most common personality disorder in clinical settings, present in 10% of all psychiatric outpatients and 15%–20% of psychiatric inpatients.

E4. _____ The diagnosis of borderline personality disorder tends to be made among females, with a female-to-male ratio of 3:1.

E5. _____ The disorder is primarily found in Western, more socioeconomically advanced countries.

E6. _____ Borderline personality disorder occurs in an estimated 2% of the general population.

E7. _____ There is no biological component to the disorder. It is typically the result of childhood traumas, especially sexual abuse.

ANSWERS: SCORING, RELATIVE WEIGHTS, AND COMMENTS

High positive scores (+3 and above) indicate a decision that would be effective, would be required for diagnosis, and without which management would be negligent. Lower positive scores (+2) indicate a decision that is important but not immediately necessary. The lowest positive score (+1) indicates a decision that is potentially useful for diagnosis and treatment. A neutral score (0) indicates a decision that is neither clearly helpful nor harmful under the given circumstances. High negative scores (−5) indicate a decision that is inappropriate and potentially harmful or possibly life-threatening. Lower negative scores (−2 and above) indicate a decision that is nonproductive and potentially harmful.

DECISION POINT A

Given this presentation, what is your differential diagnosis for axis I and axis II, according to the DSM-IV-TR criteria?

Axis I:	Axis I: Major depressive disorder (+2 points); rule out bipolar disorder type II (+2 points); polysubstance dependence (+2 points); substance-induced mood disorder (+2 points); rule out PTSD (+1 point)
Axis II:	Axis II: Mixed personality disorder (+2 points); borderline personality disorder (+2 points)

Axis I

1. **Major depressive disorder (+2).** Requirements include a 2-week history of symptoms that represent a change from previous functioning, including depressed mood or loss of interest or pleasure. In addition, patients must have at least five of nine symptoms listed in DSM-IV-TR and not meet criteria for mixed episode; symptoms cause clinically significant distress or impairment, are not due to direct physiological effects of a substance or a general medical condition, and are not better accounted for by bereavement.

   This patient has exhibited depressive symptoms on and off since her junior year in high school, when her grades began to slip and she started experimenting with drugs and alcohol. The following year, her history of suicide attempts began, and at least one of them required medical intervention to save her life. Multiple suicide attempts may also be related to bipolar disorder or borderline personality disorder rather than only to major depression.

   At the same time, the picture of major depression becomes muddled by this patient's extensive abuse of different street drugs and alcohol, which she uses to cause either unconsciousness or to allow herself to engage in extremely risky behaviors, such as extramarital affairs and disappearing for several days at a time to "party hard" without contacting friends. Consequently, it is difficult to separate the mood disorder from the substance abuse/dependence, which makes this diagnosis difficult. Once her substance use is under control, then a further assessment of her mood stability would be more appropriate and a clearer diagnosis could be made.

2. **Rule out bipolar disorder (+2).** Requires abnormally and persistently elevated, expansive, or irritable mood lasting 4 days (hypomanic-bipolar II), or 7 days (manic-bipolar I). There must also be three or more of the following: inflated self-esteem or grandiosity; decreased need for sleep; hyperverbal, pressured speech; flight of ideas, racing thoughts; distractibility; increased goal-directed activity or psychomotor agitation; and excessive involvement in pleasurable activities that have a high potential for painful consequences.

   The same caveats exist for this diagnosis as for other mood disorders. This patient certainly demonstrates grandiosity; possibly decreased need for sleep, although that was not specifically asked; distractibility in her inability to focus on school work; definite increased goal-directed activities; and excessive involvement in risky behaviors. However, many of these symptoms could be related more to substance dependence/abuse, thus muddling this diagnosis as well. She did not exhibit any of the classic symptoms of being hyperverbal and having pressured speech or racing thoughts. This does not preclude a diagnosis of bipolar disorder, but it seems her symptoms may be more related to substance and alcohol use than to an another underlying disorder. Furthermore, as stated above, removal of the alcohol and substance use would allow for a clearer picture of any underlying mood disorder.

3. **Polysubstance dependence (+2).** The patient clearly abuses a host of illicit street drugs, many of which are very dangerous as she is well aware of ("I know someone whose brain turned to mush"). She also admitted to engaging in dangerous behaviors to obtain drugs, such as sleeping with drug dealers and engaging in violent sex against her will. Her use of higher doses demonstrates tolerance to the drugs. She spends a great deal of time obtaining them, and her school and friendships have suffered as a result. She attempted to obtain alprazolam from another physician and became angry when he would not supply it, and she seems now to be attempting to get medications from you. For these reasons, it is accurate to diagnose a polysubstance dependence.

4. **Alcohol abuse (−2), alcohol dependence (−2).** For alcohol dependence, there must be physiological dependence indicated by evidence of tolerance or symptoms of withdrawal. Alcohol abuse requires fewer symptoms and may be less severe in its destructive pattern, leading to significant social, occupational, or medical impairment.

   In alcohol dependence, alcohol use is continued despite the knowledge of having a persistent or recurrent physical or psychological problem that is likely to have been worsened by alcohol (e.g., continued drinking despite knowing that an ulcer was made worse by drinking alcohol). This patient seems to be more alcohol dependent than an alcohol abuser; she did require at least two substance abuse treatment programs and relapsed shortly after each one. She drinks alone to help her sleep, and she has tried to cut down and is unable to do so. She admits to drinking three or four times per week; this is likely an underestimate, but even if it is not, it is still substantial enough for the diagnosis. In either case, however, given the totality of her substance use, she qualifies more specifically for polysubstance dependence.

5. **Substance-induced mood disorder (+2).** The key would be whether the patient's mood disorders are reversible with the cessation of her drug and alcohol use. Until she stops completely for a length of time, you will not be able to determine this. Consequently, it remains in the differential but is not conclusive.

6. **Posttraumatic stress disorder (−2).** This patient was allegedly exposed to physical, emotional, and sexual abuse as a child between the ages of 6 and 9. She has also experienced violent sexual encounters with drug dealers. As a child, she likely felt fear, helplessness, or horror as she was abused by close relatives, people to whom she looked for guidance and safety. By accusing her of causing the incidents, her mother would not emotionally validate her experiences and instead blamed her.

   The patient did not admit to recurrent and intrusive distressing recollections of the abuse events, only that they happened. After further evaluation, such an admission might be elicited, but given the information provided, you cannot assume that this will occur. She did not endorse dreams of the events or dissociative flashback episodes, and she did not express intense psychological distress when she was confronted by a presumably similar event such as being violently sexually assaulted by drug dealers as an adult. She does avoid discussing the trauma and says that she is unable to discuss it, and she became tearful when she declined to discuss it. She feels detached and estranged from others-from friends, from family, from her ex-husband. She cannot feel "loved" unless she takes Ecstasy. She has difficulty falling asleep and has difficulty concentrating. She is also prone to irritability, and reports that she yelled at her college friends "for no reason" or because they did not understand her. Although she does not endorse the hypervigilant aspects of PTSD, she does endorse enough of the other symptoms for the diagnosis to be considered.

   Hence, further investigation would be required to rule out PTSD (+1 point).

7. **Generalized anxiety disorder (−2).** This patient does not describe an inability to control anxiety or worry. She does demonstrate some of the symptoms of anxiety, such as restlessness, difficulty concentrating, irritability, and sleep disturbance, but these may all be symptomatic of substance or alcohol dependence.

8. **Substance-induced anxiety disorder (−2).** The patient does not describe panic attacks but has some anxiety symptoms. These are likely directly related to her substance and alcohol dependence.

9. **Gender identity disorder (−2).** The patient demonstrates bisexuality, not a disturbance of her gender identification.

Axis II

To have a personality disorder, a patient must have an enduring pattern of inner experience and behavior that deviates markedly from the expectations of the individual's culture in two or more of the following areas: cognition, affectivity, interpersonal, functioning, and impulse control. This patient clearly demonstrates deviations in all of these areas. She perceives others as less important than herself, she has unclear sexual preferences, and she does not appreciate the gravity of the dangerous situations into which she places herself, such as having sex with drug dealers (she thinks about what she will give them and then is surprised when they want something different). She may have been sexually harassed at her magazine job, but this is unclear as we are hearing only one side of the story. It is possible that she misconstrued her boss's behavior to suit her own mistaken impression. She is considered "moody" and has extreme swings of mood. She is emotionally labile and is prone to "freaking out" and acting inappropriately. She has difficult, tumultuous relationships with her family, friends, and ex-husband, on whom she cheated extensively. Thus she demonstrates poor impulse control in areas related to sex, drugs, and jobs.

She most closely qualifies for an axis II diagnosis in cluster B, the "dramatic emotional" type. While she does have some of the characteristics of antisocial personality disorder (failure to respect lawful behaviors, deceitfulness, impulsivity, irritability, recklessness, consistent irresponsibility), she does not carry these traits to the extent required for this diagnosis. For example, she violates the law by using illegal drugs, but she does not sell drugs, is not involved in criminal activity, and does not repeatedly perform acts that are truly grounds for arrest. Most of her antisocial behaviors involve self-inflicted harm. She is deceitful and cheats on her boyfriend, but she does not con others for personal profit. She may do so on a weak scale for personal pleasure, but she has not given any indication of a more pervasive pattern. Impulsivity is a characteristic that is nonspecific. Her reckless disregard is directed more at herself and less toward others, even if they are injured by her behaviors. Again, the behavior does not indicate the more aggressive, illegal, and conniving behavior one finds with antisocial personality disorder. Finally, consistent irresponsibility is not as clearly diagnosed in her case, and, moreover, she is able to maintain a job, maintain relationships, and maintain enough consistent behaviors at work and elsewhere that this is not the source of her major troubles.

She does demonstrate strong histrionic and narcissistic personality traits. For histrionic personality traits, she does enjoy being the center of attention, but it is not necessary for her. She is sexually provocative (including, for example, when she entered your office), and she is somewhat promiscuous. It would appear from her story that she uses her physical appearance and sexuality to draw attention to herself. She is noted to have some affected speech, but not overly so. Her presentation is definitely dramatic, and she is somewhat suggestible by others or circumstances. Finally, it seems she sees many of her relationships in black or white terms, over or under valuing relationships, considering them to be more intimate than they may be, or the opposite.

For narcissistic personality traits, she seems grandiose, inflating her self-importance and exaggerating her personal achievements. She is not preoccupied with fantasies of unlimited success, power, brilliance, beauty, or ideal love. She expresses some aspect of feeling "above others," but not to the point where she is unable to associate with anyone "beneath her" (notably when it comes to acquiring drugs). She requires admiration, but it would not seem excessively so. There is no enduring sense of entitlement and interpersonal exploitation (except with some love entanglements and perhaps to get more drugs, but these are not personality disorders but rather means to an end—which itself is related to a different psychiatric diagnosis). She is empathic but does not spend a great deal of time being envious or demonstrating arrogant haughty behaviors or attitudes. Not enough to warrant the diagnosis.

1. Thus, one possible diagnosis for the differential on axis II is **mixed personality disorder (+2).**

   The pattern of her behaviors and personality are enduring, inflexible, and pervasive across a broad range of personal and social situations. These patterns have caused disruptions in her personal, social, educational, and occupational pursuits. The onset was during childhood, and the patterns are not better accounted for by another psychiatric disorder, except perhaps drug and alcohol dependence. However, if she was raped when she was 6 to 9 years old, which preceded her first self-

destructive behaviors, we are likely to side with the personality disorder's preceding the alcohol and drug use disorders.

2. **Borderline personality disorder (+2).** The patient's personality disorder most closely follows the criteria for borderline personality disorder, as indicated by her meeting at least five of the nine DSM-IV-TR criteria:

   Frantic efforts to avoid real or imagined abandonment. She engages in multiple, often risky sexual relationships with men and women to satisfy a need to be wanted. She uses her sexuality to obtain drugs and maintain relationships with drug dealers, although, again, this is more likely a consequence of her substance dependence. She uses Ecstasy because it makes her feel "loved," which she is unable to feel among friends or family.

   Long pattern of tumultuous relationships, often characterized by extremes of idealization or devaluation. She thinks her uncle, who molested her, is smart because he's an architect, and she loves him despite the molestation. She hated her boss at the magazine and said she's an idiot. She thinks she is smarter than others and exaggerates her accomplishments, such as graduating from college magna cum laude. She at first adored her husband and then decided he was not worthy of her and sought ways to break off the relationship.

   Identity disturbance. She is not sure whether she is bisexual or heterosexual. She never fully explains what she thinks of herself, only how she reacts to others and how others are making her life more difficult.

   Impulsivity. Clearly stated impulsivity in areas that are self-damaging, such as sex and substance abuse.

   Recurrent suicidal behavior, gestures, self-mutilating behaviors.

   Affective instability due to a marked reactivity of mood in the form of "freaking out" and being known as "moody."

   Chronic feelings of emptiness-none elicited.

   Inappropriate, intense anger or difficulty controlling anger. Again, "freaking out."

   Transient, stress-related paranoid ideation or severe dissociative symptoms. "People just try to hurt me. I've never known love."

DECISION POINT B

B1. ____ +2 The statistic of 8%–10% for successful suicides is correct for borderline patients. This patient theoretically is at increased risk because of her previous attempts, and her comorbid disorders, such as alcohol and substance abuse, exacerbate the risk severalfold. Moreover, her life, personal and occupational, is very unstable. Contracting for safety has its limitations; a safety plan is of high priority. This patient could probably best benefit from dialectical behavioral therapy to help her in the long run in developing effective and safe coping strategies, regulating her emotions, and learning to tolerate stress. We cannot say, however, that her risk is definite. Determining suicide risk is not a science. Often it is the patient we think is the most safe who surprises us.

B2. ____ +3 As stated above, it is impossible to ascertain the likelihood of the patient's making another suicide attempt, but given her circumstances, risk factors, and poor social supports, it seems likely that without intervention she will try again. One intervention for which there is some empirical evidence on helping with suicidal ideation, mood stabilization, and better control of mood is dialectical behavior therapy.

B3. ____ +1 This is true. However, you should attempt a more informed assessment of her risk by asking pertinent questions, as in B4.

B4. ____ +2 This is true, and you are asking for more information to substantiate your opinion of her risk for suicide. However, this answer does not provide further steps to take.

B5. ____ +5 This is true, and beginning both dialectical behavioral therapy and substance abuse treatment, typically the latter before the former if not both at the same time, is necessary for the greatest impact on the patient's ability to develop better coping strategies, stay away from risky behaviors, and manage a hopefully more stable mood.

DECISION POINT C

According to current evidence supported by two or more randomized, placebo-controlled, doubleblind trials, what are the most effective psychopharmacological treatment recommendations for affective dysregulation symptoms, impulse-behavioral dyscontrol symptoms, and cognitive-perceptual symptoms in patients with borderline personality disorder? For each class, fill in the appropriate drugs if they meet the above mentioned evidence-based criteria. (One point is given for each correctly placed drug. Two points are deducted for incorrect answers.)

Drug Class	Affective Dysregulation Symptoms[a]	Impulse-Behavioral Dyscontrol Symptoms[b]	Cognitive-Perceptual Symptoms[c]
SSRIs and related antidepressants	Fluoxetine (+2 points) Sertraline (+2 points) Venlafaxine (+2 points)	Fluoxetine (+2 points) Sertraline (+2 points)	Agents primarily used as adjunctive treatment (+2 points)
MAOIs		Phenelzine (+2 points) Tranylcypromine (+2 points)	Agents primarily used as adjunctive treatment (+2 points)
Mood stabilizers		Lithium carbonate (+2 points) Divalproex (+2 points)	
Benzodiazepines			
Atypical antipsychotics	Olanzapine (+2 points)	Olanzapine (+2 points)	Olanzapine (+2 points)
Conventional antipsychotics	Haloperidol (+2 points)	Haloperidol (+2 points)	Haloperidol (+2 points)

SSRIs = selective serotonin reuptake inhibitors; MAOIs = monoamine oxidase inhibitors
[a]Affective dysregulation symptoms include depressed mood, mood lability, rejection sensitivity, anxiety, impulsivity, self-mutilation, anger/ hostility, psychoticism, poor global functioning, and behavioral dyscontrol.
[b]Impulse-behavioral dyscontrol symptoms include impulsive aggression, anger, irritability, self-injurious behavior, and poor global functioning.
[c]Cognitive-perceptual symptoms include ideas of reference, illusions, paranoid ideation, and associated anger/hostility.

DECISION POINT D

D1. _____ −2 A diagnosis of PTSD requires that the individual experienced, witnessed, or was confronted by an event or events that involved actual or threatened death or serious injury or a threat to the physical integrity of self or others. In addition to the experience, the individual's response must also have involved intense fear, helplessness, or horror. In children this may be expressed instead by disorganized or agitated behavior. Although this patient may have experienced sexual assault, she does not exhibit enough of the symptoms and behavioral changes for a diagnosis of PTSD, as stated below in D2.

D2. _____ +2 A diagnosis of PTSD requires the following: the traumatic event is persistently reexperienced; persistent avoidance of stimuli associated with the trauma and numbing of general responsiveness; persistent symptoms of increased arousal (not present before the trauma); duration of the disturbance is more than 1 month; and the disturbance causes clinically significant distress or impairment in social, occupational, or other important areas of functioning.

Our patient does not currently endorse any of these symptoms. In fact, she still "loves" one of her former abusers, her uncle. It is possible that she experienced PTSD as an acute syndrome earlier in her life, but she does not offer any suggestion of this. Additionally, not having been diagnosed with PTSD does not preclude the deleterious effects of early sexual assault.

DECISION POINT E

E1. _____ False. It is the most common, seen in 10% of outpatients, 15%–20% of inpatients, and 30%–60% of clinical populations with a personality disorder.

E2. _____ False. It is the most common, but see E1.

E3. _____ True.

E4. _____ True.

E5. _____ False. It is present in cultures around the world.

E6. _____ True.

E7. _____ False. It is approximately five times more common among first-degree biological relatives of those with the disorder than in the general population.

YOUR TOTAL

Decision Point	Your Score	Ideal Best Score
A		13
B		13
C		34
D		2
E		14
Total		76

KEY CLINICAL POINTS

1. Substance abuse treatment combined with dialectical behavioral therapy is the best choice for helping the patient with a personality disorder and comorbid substance abuse develop better coping strategies, stay away from risky behaviors, and manage a more stable mood.

2. Borderline personality disorder is the most common personality disorder, seen in 10% of outpatients, 15%–20% of inpatients, and 30%–60% of clinical populations with a personality disorder.

3. Borderline personality disorder patients often present with chronic suicidal ideation and multiple attempts. Between 8%–10% of people with BPD will complete suicide.

REFERENCES

American Psychiatric Association: Practice Guidelines for the Treatment of Psychiatric Disorders, Compendium 2006. Arlington VA, American Psychiatric Publishing

Frankenburg FR, Zanarini MC: Divalproex sodium treatment of women with borderline personality disorder and bipolar II disorder: a double-blind placebo-controlled pilot study. J Clin Psychiatry 2002; 63:442–446

Sadock BJ, Sadock VA: Synopsis of Psychiatry, 10th ed. Philadelphia, Lippincott Williams Wilkins, 2007

Schatzberg AF, Nemeroff CB: Essentials of Clinical Psychopharmacology 2nd Edition. Washington, DC, American Psychiatric Publishing, 2006

Shea SC: The Practical Art of Suicide Assessment. Hoboken, NJ, Wiley, 2002

Stone MH: Abnormalities of Personality: Within and Beyond the Realm of Treatment. New York, Norton, 1993

Zanarini MC, Frankenburg FR: Olanzapine treatment of female borderline personality disorder patients: a double-blind, placebo-controlled pilot study. J Clin Psychiatry 2001; 62:849–854

Here Today,
Gone Tomorrow

VIGNETTE PART 1

You are the attending physician on the psychiatry consultation-liaison service at a large tertiary care hospital. You receive a consult request from the medicine service that reads: "Patient crying, trying to get out of bed. Please evaluate for depression." You read the patient's record in the hospital database and learn that he is a 62-year-old divorced man who was admitted to the hospital 1 month ago for a below-the-knee amputation of his left leg, which had been gangrenous. He has severe type 2 diabetes mellitus, and he has not adhered to his medication regimen. Since the amputation he has had "mental status changes" and been treated repeatedly with 5 mg i.m. of haloperidol. He developed aspiration pneumonia during his second week in the hospital and has had three urinary tract infections since admission. He has a sacral decubitus ulcer that is being treated with piperacillin, tazobactam, and gentamycin. He has lost 65 pounds since admission. His medical history is significant for hypertension, treated with 50 mg b.i.d. of atenolol and 0.2 mg b.i.d. of clonidine. His last transesophageal echocardiogram revealed a hypokinetic left ventricle, hypertrophic right ventricle, and an ejection fraction of 20%. He had a four-vessel coronary artery bypass graft 3 years ago after a myocardial infarction. The patient has chronic obstructive pulmonary disease from 80 pack-years of smoking, and obstructive sleep apnea was diagnosed 10 years ago. He has long refused to use a continuous positive airway pressure machine at night because he is "claustrophobic."

The most recent physical examination revealed the patient to have a ruddy complexion. A nasal cannula was being used, delivering 3 liters of oxygen per minute. His heart rate was regular at 108 bpm, and his blood pressure was 197/100. He had a temperature of 99.5°F, treated 1 hour ago with 800 mg of acetaminophen. He had jugular venous distention at approximately 5 cm, S3 could be appreciated, and a 2/6 systolic murmur in the upper right sternal border and bilateral wheezing on auscultation of the chest could be heard. The patient had 2–3+ pitting edema on his right lower extremity to the knee. His left lower extremity above the knee incision was mildly erythematous, weeping clear fluid in three places where the incision was slightly dehisced. The examination was otherwise unremarkable.

The patient's most recent lab results, from that morning, were as follows:

CBC: wbc 16.8, hem 10.8, hct 31.4, plt 82
BASIC: Na 127, K 2.4, Cl 99, HCO3 28, Cr 3.2, BUN 148, GLU 188
COMP: Cal 9.7, Alb 3.2, Prot 5.4, AST 26, ALT 22, Alk Phos 177
Urinalysis: leukocyte esterase positive, nitrite positive, wbc > 25 per hpf, rbc 2–5 per hpf, hyaline casts 2–3 per hpf
Urine drug screen: positive for opiates, benzodiazepines
Oxygen saturation was 92% on 3 liters via nasal cannula
Chest X-ray showed enlarged heart silhouette, bilateral pleural effusion, no signs of infectious process; evidence of previous open heart surgery.

DECISION POINT A

Given this history, list the top five issues for this patient that could result in delirium or could exacerbate a delirium. (Check your responses against the list provided in the Answers section. Points are awarded for all correct responses specifically relating to this patient.)

1.

2.

3.

4.

5.

VIGNETTE PART 2

At 7:30 p.m. you are paged by the medicine intern, who wishes to speak with you urgently. You call back and he reports that the patient has pulled out his IV and his Foley catheter. The patient struck two nurses and then a security guard with closed fists as they placed him in four-point restraints. The patient is now stiffening, his head is turning to the side, his tongue looks thickened, he is "making crazy faces," and he is unable to respond to any external stimuli. The intern is very anxious and wants advice on how to manage this patient. He wants to know if it was appropriate to put the patient into restraints and whether to administer haloperidol.

DECISION POINT B

Based on this information, your next step should include which of the following? (More than one answer is possible. Points are taken away for incorrect answers. Answers should be prioritized.)

B1. _____ Tell the intern that the patient is very likely "sundowning" and that the most appropriate step would be to give him 10 mg i.m. haloperidol immediately. Tell him that you will be there shortly to assess the patient and make further recommendations.

B2. _____ Tell the intern that the patient is likely "sundowning" and that the best course of action is to reorient him, maintain him in four-point restraints, and administer 2 mg of lorazepam intramuscularly or orally every 4 hours for agitation.

B3. _____ Tell the intern that the description of the patient suggests that he is suffering an acute dystonia, likely secondary to the large doses of haloperidol. Tell him that you will be there shortly, but he should immediately give the patient 50 mg i.v. of diphenhydramine. Tell him that an anticholinergic agent could worsen the delirium but that because patients can develop laryngeal dystonia, treatment is necessary. Tell him to remove the restraints as soon as the patient calms down.

B4. _____ Tell the intern that the patient probably has a CNS infection and should be transferred immediately to the intensive care unit. Tell him that an intravenous haloperidol drip of 0.2 mg per hour should be started and a lumbar puncture performed and that empirical treatment of bacterial meningitis should be considered while the patient's cerebrospinal fluid is evaluated.

B5. _____ Tell the intern that the patient should be placed in a Posey restraint as well as the four-point leather restraints to keep him in bed. Tell him that there is no treatment for this condition and that the patient must "ride it out." Assure him that this episode will be over within 4–6 hours.

VIGNETTE PART 3

You check the patient's current medications list, which includes the following:

1. Glyburide 5 mg p.o. daily
2. Metformin 500 mg p.o. b.i.d.
3. Insulin sliding scale with Humalog
4. Aspirin 81 mg p.o. daily
5. Furosemide 160 mg p.o. daily
6. Piperacillin/tazobactam 3.375 grams i.v. every 6 hours
7. Gentamycin 2 grams i.v. every 8 hours
8. Atenolol 50 mg p.o. b.i.d.
9. Lisinopril 20 mg p.o. daily
10. Clonidine 0.2 mg p.o. b.i.d.
11. Fluoxetine 60 mg p.o. daily
12. Fluticasone/salmeterol 5/500 2 puffs b.i.d.
13. Albuterol 2 puffs b.i.d.
14. Haloperidol 10 mg p.o. or i.m. every 6 hours p.r.n. for agitation (total 40 mg in 3 days)
15. Trazodone 200 mg p.o. h.s.
16. Zolpidem 10 mg p.o. h.s.

DECISION POINT C

Given the patient's presentation and this list of medications, specify your degree of concern regarding drug interactions or direct adverse effects for each medication. (Scoring is individualized to each drug. Identify your level of concern in terms of the medication causing or exacerbating a delirium. Your choices are "No concern," "Possibly dangerous," or "Definitely dangerous." Points are taken away for incorrect answers.)

Medication	No Concern	Possibly Dangerous	Definitely Dangerous
C1. Glyburide			
C2. Metformin			
C3. Insulin sliding scale with Humalog			
C4. Aspirin			
C5. Furosemide			
C6. Piperacillin/tazobactam			
C7. Gentamycin			
C8. Atenolol			
C9. Lisinopril			
C10. Clonidine			
C11. Fluoxetine			
C12. Fluticasone/salmeterol			
C13. Albuterol			
C14. Haloperidol p.r.n.			
C15. Trazodone			
C16. Zolpidem			

DECISION POINT D

What is the most likely predisposing factor for delirium in this patient?

D1. _____ Numerous new medications starting during the hospitalization

D2. _____ Any iatrogenic event

D3. _____ Use of a bladder catheter

D4. _____ Visual impairment

D5. _____ None of the above

DECISION POINT E

Because antipsychotics and serotonergic agents are both used in treating delirium, the severe side effects of neuroleptic malignant syndrome, serotonin syndrome, or extrapyramidal side effects should be considered in this case. Match the following symptoms or signs with the appropriate diagnosis. (More than one answer may apply to each symptom or sign. One point is given for correct signs and symptoms. Points are taken away for incorrect responses.)

Sign or Symptom	Extrapyramidal Side Effects	Serotonin Syndrome	Neuroleptic Malignant Syndrome
E1. Mental status changes			
E2. Behavioral-restlessness or agitation			
E3. Autonomic dysfunction			
E4. Physical examination			
a. Myoclonus			
b. Hyperreflexia			
c. Tremor			
d. Incoordination			
e. Muscle rigidity			
f. Trismus			
g. Blepharospasm			
h. Oculogyric crisis			
i. Dysarthria			
j. Dysphagia			
E5. Laboratory values			
a. Elevated creatinine phosphokinase			
b. Leukocytosis			
c. Myoglobinuria			
d. Metabolic acidosis			

DECISION POINT F

Patients who exhibit difficulty concentrating can be misdiagnosed as having delirium, dementia, and major depression. Match the following symptoms and signs as related to delirium, dementia, or major depression. (Points are given for positive answers. Each symptom can have more than one correct answer, so mark as many as you think apply. Points are taken away for incorrect answers.)

Symptom or Sign	Delirium	Dementia	Major Depression
F1. Memory impairment is early sign			
F2. Aphasia, apraxia, agnosia, or disturbance in executive functioning			
F3. Acute onset			
F4. Poor judgment, poor insight			
F5. Difficulty with spatial tasks			
F6. Disturbance of consciousness			
F7. Disturbance of attention			
F8. Disturbance of cognition			
F9. Disturbance of perception			
F10. Marked fluctuation during the course of the day			

ANSWERS: SCORING, RELATIVE WEIGHTS, AND COMMENTS

High positive scores (+3 and above) indicate a decision that would be effective, would be required for diagnosis, and without which management would be negligent. Lower positive scores (+2) indicate a decision that is important but not immediately necessary. The lowest positive score (+1) indicates a decision that is potentially useful for diagnosis and treatment. A neutral score (0) indicates a decision that is neither clearly helpful nor harmful under the given circumstances. High negative scores (−3 and above) indicate a decision that is inappropriate and potentially harmful or life-threatening. Lower negative scores (−2) indicate a decision that is nonproductive and potentially harmful. The lowest negative score (−1) indicates a decision that is not harmful but is nonproductive, time-consuming, and not cost-effective.

DECISION POINT A

A1. ____ +5 History: Determine what the patient's baseline mental status was prior to admission. Has the patient had previous bouts of mental status changes? If so, what was done?

A2. ____ +5 Psychiatric conditions: The patient was described as "depressed." Does he have a preexisting psychiatric condition? Has he ever been on any psychotropic medications?

A3. ____ +5 Medications: What medications is the patient currently taking? What medications was the patient taking prior to admission? Check for drug-drug interactions and iatrogenic causes.

A4. ____ +5 Substances/alcohol: The patient's urine drug screen was positive for opiates and benzodiazepines. Does the patient have a history of abuse or dependence on alcohol or other substances? Is the patient within the window of withdrawal from any of the possible offending agents?

A5. ____ +5 Endocrine: Is the patient eating adequately while receiving treatment for diabetes? Is this renal failure or liver failure? Are endocrine abnormalities possible, such as hypo- or hyperthyroidism or hypo- or hyperparathyroidism?

A6. ____ +5 Metabolic: Could the delirium be secondary to a thiamine or other nutritional deficiency? Is there an acid-base disturbance? Could the patient be in heart failure?

A7. ____ +5 Vascular: The patient is hypertensive. Could he have hypertensive encephalopathy? Cerebral arteriosclerosis? Could he have cardiac emboli from atrial fibrillation? Patent foramen ovale? Endocarditic valve?

A8. ____ +5 Infectious: Does the patient have a urinary tract infection? Obtain a urinalysis with culture and susceptibility, and also look at the urine to see if it is clear or cloudy. Given the patient's multiple sources of infection, it is reasonable to pan-culture the patient's infectious sources. Is he becoming septic/encephalitic/meningitic from bacteria or virus? He is less likely to have a parasitic or fungal infection, but this may need to be ruled out given the possibility of immunocompromise from multiple medical problems. The patient has multiple sources of possible infection, with a dehisced amputation wound, pneumonia or other lung infection, septic joint, sacral decubitus ulcer, and so on.

A9. _____ +5 Brain hypoxia: Could the patient have brain hypoxia secondary to cardiac insufficiency, pulmonary infection, or chronic obstructive pulmonary disease? Could anemia be causing the delirium?

DECISION POINT B

B1. _____ −5 You do not know how much haloperidol the patient has received to this point. Moreover, the patient's symptoms sound like acute dystonic reaction, an extrapyramidal side effect. You do not wish to worsen these symptoms, so it makes sense to back off the haloperidol and give a trial of 50 mg i.v. of diphenhydramine or 1–2 mg i.v. of benztropine to see if the symptoms abate. If the symptoms continue unchanged or worsen, then other causes must be explored, especially a CNS infection.

B2. _____ −3 First, perform a bedside neurological exam and a Mini-Mental State Examination to establish a current baseline. Data are limited on the efficacy of benzodiazepines for the treatment of delirium, except in the case of alcohol or benzodiazepine withdrawal. Although there are reports of successful use of a combination of a benzodiazepine and an antipsychotic in treating delirium, these reports are inconclusive and did not use standardized assessment tools. Benzodiazepines can increase sedation and cause behavioral inhibition, amnesia, ataxia, respiratory depression, physical dependence, rebound insomnia, withdrawal reactions, and delirium. Lorazepam, oxazepam, and temazepam are primarily metabolized by glucuronidation, not oxidated, and clonazepam is acetylated. Thus, all are rela-

tively unaffected until parenchymal liver disease is quite severe; they are subsequently relatively safer in the context of liver failure if a benzodiazepine is necessary to treat withdrawal symptoms, to raise seizure threshold, or to counteract anticholinergic side effects or akathisia associated with concurrent use of antipsychotics. For this patient, whose medical history includes extensive lung disease, obstructive sleep apnea, chronic renal insufficiency, and hepatic encephalopathy, benzodiazepines are relatively contraindicated.

B3. _____ +3 Because this seems a likely cause of the current classical manifestation of an extrapyramidal acute dystonic reaction (thickened tongue, stiffening, torticollis, and facial grimacing), a small trial of an anticholinergic is reasonable. Anticholinergics, antiparkinsonian agents, and antihistamines such as trihexyphenidyl, benztropine, biperiden, procyclidine, and diphenhydramine are all commonly used for the treatment of neuroleptic-induced parkinsonism and acute dystonic reactions. Diphenhydramine can be given up to a total of 400 mg/day. Keep in mind that you have not yet seen the patient and may be surprised when you get to the bedside. Typically in these circumstances the patient must be reevaluated frequently, and physical restraints should be removed once the patient is considered safe from harm to himself or others.

B4. _____ +2 A CNS infection is lower on the differential diagnosis but must still be considered, especially if the more likely scenario of acute dystonic reaction secondary to antipsychotic use is ruled out. If suspicion of a CNS infection rises, computed tomography of the head and a lumbar puncture are indicated, in which case the patient will likely require sedation to lie still through the procedures.

B5. _____ −5 This response is inappropriate in a hospital. Patients' comfort and safety must be maintained, and this patient's condition is very likely treatable and not something to "ride out."

DECISION POINT C

Assign +1 point for each correct answer, and −1 point for each incorrect answer. Explanation follows the table.

Medication	No Concern	Possibly Dangerous	Definitely Dangerous
C1. Glyburide			X
C2. Metformin			X
C3. Insulin sliding scale with Humalog			X
C4. Aspirin		X	
C5. Furosemide		X	
C6. Piperacillin/tazobactam			X
C7. Gentamycin		X	
C8. Atenolol	X		
C9. Lisinopril		X	
C10. Clonidine		X	
C11. Fluoxetine		X	
C12. Fluticasone/salmeterol		X	
C13. Albuterol	X		
C14. Haloperidol p.r.n.			X
C15. Trazodone			X
C16. Zolpidem		X	

EXPLANATION FOR DECISION POINT C

1. Drug-drug interactions

   a. Fluoxetine-trazodone: May result in toxic levels of either fluoxetine (serotonin syndrome, including hypertension, hyperthermia, myoclonus, and mental status changes) or trazodone (sedation, dry mouth, urinary retention)

   b. Haloperidol-fluoxetine: May exacerbate the side effects of the antipsychotic, including pseudoparkinsonism, akathisia, tongue stiffness, increased risk of cardiotoxicity (QT interval prolongation, torsade de pointes, and cardiac arrest)

2. Disease contraindications

   a. Hydrochlorothiazide/lisinopril: Hyperglycemia, hyperuricemia

   b. Furosemide: Hyperglycemia, hyperuricemia

   c. Clonidine: Hyperglycemia, hyperuricemia

3. General

   a. Piperacillin/tazobactam must be renally calculated given the patient's poor kidney function.

   b. Zolpidem: This drug is known to cause worsening mental status in certain people, especially the elderly.

c. The inhalers are helping the patient breathe and do not have any drug-drug interactions or contraindications in this patient.

d. Insulin sliding scale: This should be carefully monitored according to the patient's appetite, blood glucose chemsticks, and testing. If the patient will not be eating, either for testing or because of lack of appetite, the insulin scale must be carefully monitored so as not to allow him to become hypo- or hyperglycemic, which could result in a change in mental status.

DECISION POINT D

D1. _____ +4 Multiple medications are always a concern in the development of a delirium. Of particular concern are medications with anticholinergic effects. When several of these medications are started, an anticholinergic delirium is more likely to occur.

D2. _____ 0 An iatrogenic event does not necessarily put the patient at risk for a delirium.

D3. _____ +1 An indwelling catheter puts patients at risk of developing a bladder infection and subsequent sepsis. In elderly patients the first sign of sepsis may be a change in mental status.

D4. _____ +2 Impairment of vision and/or hearing places patients at risk of developing a delirium.

Other risk factors that should, if present, cause the clinician to assume delirium is present until proven otherwise include:

1. Advanced age (especially over 80 years)
2. Severe illness (especially cancer)
3. Dehydration
4. Dementia
5. Fever or hypothermia
6. Substance abuse
7. Azotemia
8. Hypoalbuminemia
9. Abnormal sodium levels

DECISION POINT E

More than one answer may apply to each symptom or sign. One point is given for necessary signs or symptoms, and 2 points if the sign or symptom is a necessary criterion for diagnosis (these are indicated by two X's). Points are taken away for incorrect responses.

Sign or Symptom	Extrapyramidal Side Effects	Serotonin Syndrome	Neuroleptic Malignant Syndrome
E1. Mental status changes		X	X
E2. Behavioral-restlessness or agitation	X	X	X
E3 Autonomic dysfunction			XX
E4. Physical examination			
a. Myoclonus	X	X	X
b. Hyperreflexia	X	X	X
c. Tremor	X	X	X
d. Incoordination		X	
e. Muscle rigidity	X	X	XX
f. Trismus	X		
g. Blepharospasm	X		
h. Oculogyric crisis	X		
i. Dysarthria	X		
j. Dysphagia	X		
E5. Laboratory values			
a. Elevated creatinine phosphokinase			X
b. Leukocytosis			X
c. Myoglobinuria			X
d. Metabolic acidosis			X

DECISION POINT F

Patients who exhibit difficulty concentrating can be misdiagnosed as having delirium, dementia, and major depression. Match the following symptoms and signs as related to delirium, dementia, or major depression. (Points are given for positive answers. Each symptom can have more than one correct answer, so mark as many as you think apply. Points are taken away for incorrect answers.)

Symptom or Sign	Delirium	Dementia	Major Depression
F1. Memory impairment is early sign	X	X	
F2. Aphasia, apraxia, agnosia, or disturbance in executive functioning	X	X	
F3. Acute onset	X		
F4. Poor judgment, poor insight	X	X	
F5. Difficulty with spatial tasks	X	X	
F6. Disturbance of consciousness	X		
F7. Disturbance of attention	X	X	X
F8. Disturbance of cognition	X	X	X
F9. Disturbance of perception	X	X	
F10. Marked fluctuation during the course of the day	X		

KEY CLINICAL POINTS

1. An accurate diagnosis of dementia requires thoroughly ruling out other similar presenting disorders such as depression, substance abuse, physical causes or medications ingested.
2. Psychoactive medications commonly used without incident in a younger adult population may have serious adverse effects in an older population presenting with dementia.
3. Delirium is a common and potentially fatal confounding condition that must be differentiated from dementia.

YOUR TOTAL

Decision Point	Your Score	Ideal Best Score
A		25
B		5
C		16
D		7
E		30
F		19
Total		102

REFERENCES

American Psychiatric Association: Practice Guidelines for the Treatment of Psychiatric Disorders, Compendium 2006. Arlington, VA, American Psychiatric Publishing

Inouye SK: A practical program for preventing delirium in hospitalized elderly patients. Cleve Clin J Med 2004; 71:890–896

Mitchell A J. A meta-analysis of the accuracy of the mini-mental state examination in the detection of dementia and mild cognitive impairment. Journal of Psychiatric Research 2009; 43(4): 411–431

Rodda J, Morgan S, Walker Z. Are cholinesterase inhibitors effective in the management of the behavioral and psychological symptoms of dementia in Alzheimer's disease? A systematic review of randomized, placebo-controlled trials of donepezil, rivastigmine and galantamine. International Psychogeriatrics 2009; 21(5): 813–824

Sadock BJ, Sadock VA: Synopsis of Psychiatry, 10th ed. Philadelphia, Lippincott Williams & Wilkins, 2007

Schatzberg AF, Nemeroff CB: Textbook of Psychopharmacology. Arlington VA, American Psychiatric Publishing, 2009

Wyszynski AA, Wyszynski B: Manual of Psychiatric Care for the Medically Ill. Arlington, Va, American Psychiatric Publishing, 2005

Scheduling Time to Raise the 'Perfect' Daughter

VIGNETTE PART 1

You are a child psychiatrist at a large medical center and occasionally take weekend call from home for the psychiatric emergency room. You receive an urgent phone call at 8:00 p.m. from the psychiatric emergency room resident. Ms. A, a 14-year-old ninth-grade student at a prestigious private all-girl school, is there, accompanied by her parents. According to the resident, Ms. A admits to taking "a big handful" of aspirin two nights earlier but did not tell anyone and was not treated. Tonight, after she had made superficial cuts on her right wrist with a razor blade, her parents brought her to the emergency department. Because the cuts did not require sutures, the attending emergency physician transferred her to the psychiatric emergency room for evaluation. The patient's parents insist that their daughter is probably just worried about her end-of-year exams and is otherwise fine and that she needs to go home. The psychiatric resident feels that the girl is ambivalent about being suicidal, and he is not convinced that she is safe to go home. He is calling to ask for your opinion on whether Ms. A should be admitted.

DECISION POINT A

Given this history, which of the following would you do? (Select the best answer.)

A1. _____ Ask to speak with the parents. Tell them that they are probably right about their daughter's anxiety and should take her home for the night, then bring her to your office tomorrow after school for an appointment.

A2. _____ Ask to speak with the parents. Tell them you cannot assess their daughter from home and that you are deferring to the judgment of the resident, who thinks their daughter should be admitted for safety.

A3. _____ Ask to speak with the parents. Tell them their daughter is not at great risk of suicide, that the cutting was merely a gesture. Tell them it is okay to take her home and tell them to call your secretary in the morning and make an appointment for sometime within the week.

A4. _____ Refuse to speak with the parents. Tell the resident that you agree the patient should be admitted for safety. Ask him to politely tell the parents that they may call you tomorrow at your office to discuss the case.

A5. _____ Refuse to speak with the parents. Speaking with the parents will only intensify Ms. A's feelings of mistrust.

VIGNETTE PART 2

Ms. A is admitted to the hospital's child and adolescent psychiatry locked ward and placed on close observation. The resident explained to the parents that you, as the attending psychiatrist, would see her the following morning. Because they were in a hurry to go home and did not know whether they would be available to come in early the next day to sign consent forms, the resident sought consent for use of several medications that you might wish to prescribe for their daughter, depending on your evaluation. They agreed and anxiously signed consent forms for use of fluoxetine, lorazepam, ziprasidone, and chlorpromazine.

You visit Ms. A the next morning. During your interview with her, she speaks slowly and has poor eye contact. She reports that she feels "depressed" and "angry with her parents." You ask her why, and she replies, "They have unreasonable expectations of me. They never let me do what I want to do. They just keep grounding me for every little thing." She is tearful and her voice becomes louder. You note that her fists are clenched tightly. You ask how she is doing in school. She responds that she gets "B's mostly, a couple of A's." You ask about other activities. She says that she is on the school soccer team, takes extra French lessons outside of school, and has taken piano lessons since age 4 and that her mother recently encouraged her to volunteer at the hospital's oncology department. At this, her eyes well up with tears: "I hate working in the hospital," she says. "Those patients, they're are all just dying, and it makes me want to die too. I hate my life."

She reports that she has been sleeping "a lot" and as a result has fallen behind on some of her school assignments, which is unlike her. She says that she used to like all of the activities and schoolwork, but now "everything is such a chore. I feel like blowing it all off just to piss off my parents." She has lost about 10 pounds in the past 2 months without dieting or changing her routine. She says that her appetite is less than it usually is and she doesn't know why, other than that she is "too busy feeling like my life is crappy and I'd rather not live." She says it has been more difficult for her to stay focused on her schoolwork over the past month and she has to try harder to accomplish the same tasks that she once found easy.

You ask how often she has thought about killing herself, and she replies that she thinks about it every day. She tells you that she recently took "a big handful" of aspirin. It made her sick to her stomach, but she did not tell anyone. "My parents grounded me when I didn't make the varsity soccer team, too." She shows you her right wrist, which is bandaged. "I didn't cut deep enough. That was stupid."

DECISION POINT B

Given this presentation, what is your next step? (Rank the following in the order in which you would perform them. Points are taken away for incorrect answers.)

B1. _____ Ask if she has ever used drugs or alcohol.

B2. _____ Ask if anyone in her family has any psychiatric problems.

B3. _____ Ask if her schoolwork is too hard for her. Determine whether she is developmentally appropriate for her grade level.

B4. _____ Ask if she has mood swings often and if she has bad premenstrual symptoms.

B5. _____ Ask if there is any suicidal ideation or specific plan to kill herself.

B6. _____ Order lab work to obtain a thyroid-stimulating hormone level, CBC, blood chemistry profile (CHEM-7), and a urine drug screen.

B7. _____ Ask if she is sexually active and determine her level of sexual behavior.

DECISION POINT C

You make a preliminary diagnosis of a mood disorder. In children and adolescents, which of the following symptoms of depression is less likely to be considered in the diagnostic criteria for adult depression? (Rank as many as appropriate, in order of their likelihood.)

C1. _____ Loss of interest or pleasure

C2. _____ Sadness

C3. _____ Emptiness

C4. _____ Irritability

C5. _____ Hypersomnolence

DECISION POINT D

When reviewing the important symptoms of depression, "SIGECAPS" is a helpful mnemonic. In the following, match each letter with the word it represents. (Answers may be used once, more than once, or not at all.)

D1. _____ S
D2. _____ I
D3. _____ G
D4. _____ E
D5. _____ C
D6. _____ A
D7. _____ P
D8. _____ S

a. _____ Ideation (suicidal or homicidal)
b. _____ Paucity of speech
c. _____ Interest (decreased)
d. _____ Excessive or disproportionate guilt
e. _____ Intellectual deficits
f. _____ Energy level
g. _____ Sleep
h. _____ Psychomotor agitation or retardation
i. _____ Excitability
j. _____ Altered consciousness
k. _____ Substance use
l. _____ Concentration
m. _____ Appetite
n. _____ Gregariousness
o. _____ Cognition
p. _____ Suicidal ideation
q. _____ Somnolence

VIGNETTE PART 3

You are paged by the desk clerk. Ms. A's mother has arrived and has brought a knapsack containing a laptop computer for her daughter. She tells you that "it is imperative" that her daughter get the computer so that she won't fall behind in her schoolwork. She remarks that "this sort of thing has been going on lately with her. I don't know why she feels the need to pull these stunts except to hurt us." She holds out the knapsack for you to take. "I really must be going," she says. "My husband is double-parked."

DECISION POINT E

Given this information, how do you respond? (Rank as many as appropriate, in order of their likelihood. Points are taken away for incorrect answers.)

E1. _____ Tell the mother that you would be happy to deliver the computer to her daughter and that she should hurry, because the police in this area love to write tickets.

E2. _____ Tell the mother that you would be happy to deliver the computer to her daughter, but that you want to speak with her and her husband about what happened.

E3. _____ Tell the mother that you cannot deliver the computer to her daughter because the ward has a policy against bringing in electronic devices, including laptop computers, for safety reasons. None of the children have them.

E4. _____ Tell the mother that you are concerned about her running off so quickly when her daughter has just tried to kill herself. Would she like to talk about it?

E5. _____ Tell the mother that you are concerned about her daughter, but that she is now in a safe place. Strongly suggest a meeting between you and both parents so you can determine what caused their daughter to make an attempt on her life twice in one week.

E6. _____ Ask the mother if she could meet with you now. Tell her to have her husband park the car properly and meet you in your office in 15 minutes. Her daughter has made a serious attempt on her life, and she should not leave without discussing the matter.

E7. _____ Ask the mother for consent to treat her daughter and, as applicable in your state, for specific consents for psychotropic medications and releases to speak with her pediatrician and her psychiatrist.

VIGNETTE PART 4

After 2 days on the ward, your patient feels more relaxed. She occasionally smiles, and she interacts with the other patients, but she still has a somewhat restricted affect. She begins complaining that she is not getting her schoolwork done and that "my parents are going to kill me." She denies that she is currently suicidal but cannot rule it out for the future. She is still sleeping excessively and did not make it to her morning group session, which kept her from advancing up the scale of earned privileges on the ward. She complains that she wants to go outside and is frustrated that she can't. She no longer wants to talk about "my problems" and asks, "Is that all I'm going to do here? Talk about problems? Why do you think I have problems? Talk to my parents They're the ones with problems!"

You later ask her about substance use, and she admits to having tried marijuana and beer in the past but insists that it is not a problem for her. "Everyone does it," she says. "I mean at parties. I'll have a beer or two, not enough to get trashed like some of my friends. My parents would kill me if I came home drunk. And I don't like pot. I don't like how it makes me feel."

DECISION POINT F

Given this information, what are your next steps? (Rank as many as appropriate in order of their likelihood. Points are taken away for incorrect answers):

F1. _____ Agree that she is not likely using drugs or alcohol in a way that is dangerous and leave this subject alone for now. Instead, concentrate on peer relationships and how they affect her own decision making.

F2. _____ Agree that she is not likely using drugs or alcohol in a way that is dangerous and leave this subject alone for now. Instead, scold her gently for not attending all of her group sessions and tell her that she will not be able to leave the ward until she improves her behavior.

F3. _____ Send for a urine drug screen if this has not already been done. If the urine drug screen is positive for any drugs, consider placing Ms. A in a discovery group or a similar group that helps young teens learn about drugs, the dangers of their use, and how to avoid being in situations where drug use might occur.

F4. _____ If the urine drug screen is positive for any drugs, do not tell Ms. A's parents. This information is entirely confidential, and revealing it might destroy the therapeutic bond with your patient.

F5. _____ If the urine drug screen is positive for any drugs, have the social services department invite Ms. A's family in to discuss alcohol and/or drug abuse and treatment options and other issues.

DECISION POINT G

Depressed patients who exhibit difficulty concentrating can be misdiagnosed as having attention deficit hyperactivity disorder (ADHD). Match the following symptoms and signs with depression, ADHD, both, or neither. (Your score will be determined by the number of questions for which "both" is the correct answer.)

Symptom or Sign	Depression	ADHD	Both	Neither
G1. Often fails to give close attention to details or makes careless mistakes in schoolwork, work, or other activities				
G2. Often does not seem to listen when spoken to directly				
G3. Increase in goal-directed activity (either socially, at work or school, or sexually)				
G4. Is often forgetful in daily activities				
G5. Insomnia or hypersomnia nearly every day				
G6. Markedly diminished interest or pleasure in all, or almost all, activities				
G7. Often loses things necessary for tasks or activities (e.g., toys, school assignments, pencils, books, or tools)				
G8. Psychomotor agitation				
G9. Inflated self-esteem or grandiosity				
G10. Often has difficulty organizing tasks and activities				

ANSWERS: SCORING, RELATIVE WEIGHTS, AND COMMENTS

High positive scores (+3 and above) indicate a decision that would be effective, would be required for diagnosis, and without which management would be negligent. Lower positive scores (+2) indicate a decision that is important but not immediately necessary. The lowest positive score (+1) indicates a decision that is potentially useful for diagnosis and treatment. A neutral score (0) indicates a decision that is neither clearly helpful nor harmful under the given circumstances. High negative scores (−3 and above) indicate a decision that is inappropriate and potentially harmful or possibly life-threatening. Lower negative scores (−2) indicate a decision that is nonproductive and potentially harmful. The lowest negative score (−1) indicates a decision that is not harmful but is nonproductive, time-consuming, and not cost-effective.

DECISION POINT A

A1. _____ +2 Although it is not necessary for the attending psychiatrist on call to speak directly with a patient or the patient's parents, you should consider doing so if they wish to speak with you or if you find that the resident and/or social worker was unable to establish a suitable rapport for assessing the situation. In this exercise, the parents are allegedly quite upset, do

not fully comprehend the gravity of their daughter's suicide attempt, and may be making matters worse for their daughter by fighting with the treatment team. Telling them that they are right about their daughter's anxiety would be inappropriate at this juncture because you do not know the current situation firsthand; however, you can offer reassurance, reflect back to them their frustration with their child's behavior, and help them better understand the issue of suicide and the need to take it seriously. The child should certainly be seen right away, but judging whether she should be admitted has less to do with the temper of her parents than the assessment of her mental status, the seriousness of her suicidal intention, and her overall safety. If she is deemed safe to go home, then her parents should closely monitor her overnight and follow up with you the next day. If she is not deemed safe to go home, then she should be admitted.

A2. _____ +5 The resident is your proxy and you must put your faith in his judgment of whether or not this child is safe. If the resident feels the child is at risk of harming herself, then she should be admitted. Speaking with the parents would be appropriate. You could also consider coming in to the hospital to obtain information firsthand.

A3. _____ −5 The resident feels that the child is not safe. You should trust his judgment or come in to the hospital to see the child yourself and discuss her situation with the psychiatric emergency room team. Waiting a week to see this patient would not be appropriate.

A4. _____ −2 While it would be appropriate to admit the patient, refusing to speak with her parents if they ask to talk with you would seem insulting to them and damage your hopes of gaining their trust. After all, you are admitting their daughter to a psychiatric ward because of a suicidal gesture they do not fully comprehend or appreciate.

A5. _____ −5 The parents may be agitated, but you should talk with them, because they may be confused about their daughter's psychiatric condition. Furthermore, given that the resident feels that the child will require admission, waiting until your next open appointment would not be appropriate.

DECISION POINT B

B1. _____ +4 Children, especially adolescents, are often experimenting with, abusing, or dependent on drugs and/or alcohol, and a mood disorder is often comorbid with the substance use disorder. Although determining which came first can be a puzzle, knowing about the substance use will help you arrive at an appropriate diagnosis and determine the best course of treatment. When a substance use problem is present, it should be treated in order to remove it as an obstacle to the patient's recovery from the mood disorder. Whether or not this patient is currently using alcohol or drugs, she has admitted to prior use.

B2. _____ +3 This is always a good question to ask, because mood disorders and other psychiatric conditions are inheritable.

B3. _____ −2 Asking if here courses are too hard for her would quickly cast you in the role of another parental figure who doesn't understand her. Earning B's and A's in classes, learning French, taking piano, and volunteering clearly indicate a high level of achievement (perhaps overachieving).

B4. _____ +2 Ms. A is at the age when she should be menstruating, and hormonal changes can cause or contribute to mood disturbances. This information should be obtained as part of your evaluation, but it is secondary to issues of safety, including suicide and substance abuse.

B5. _____ +5 This is the most important area of assessment and should guide treatment planning. High-risk indicators for continuing risk of suicide include the following:

1. The patient presents immediately after committing a serious suicidal act.
2. The patient is displaying dangerous psychotic symptoms suggestive of a high suicide risk.
3. The patient mentions suicidal planning or intent in the interview, suggesting that he or she is seriously planning imminent suicide (or corroborative sources supply information suggestive of such planning).

B6. _____ +4 Standard of care

B7. _____ +4 This is an important line of questioning with any adolescent female, particularly when considering the use of psychotropic medications. Could she be pregnant? Additionally, you want to know if there is any history of sexual, emotional, or physical abuse.

DECISION POINT C

C1. _____ 0 points
C2. _____ 0 points
C3. _____ 0 points
C4. _____ 5 points
C5. _____ 0 points

DECISION POINT D

D1. _____ +2 points g Sleep
D2. _____ +2 points c Interest
D3. _____ +2 points d Excessive guilt
D4. _____ +2 points f Energy level
D5. _____ +2 points l Concentration
D6. _____ +2 points m Appetite
D7. _____ +2 points h Psychomotor agitation
D8. _____ +2 points p Suicidal ideation

DECISION POINT E

E1. _____ −5 The patient was admitted to the ward because of a suicide attempt. She is there to recover from the event, to learn from it, to be further evaluated by the team, and to participate in group and individual milieu activities-not to continue with her schoolwork. Considering the story, it is regrettable that the mother is insistent about this issue. She should be told that it is not in her daughter's best interest to focus on schoolwork right now and that the family needs to understand what is going on in terms of the recent suicide attempts.

E2. _____ −3 You will not give the computer to the patient (as explained above), but you do want to speak with her parents.

E3. _____ +3 This would be an appropriate response. You would want to make an effort at this point to arrange to speak with the parents at some point in the near future, not necessarily at that moment.

E4. _____ +1 Although you may think this, you should be careful not to draw the mother into a confrontation about the suicidal behavior. You should assume that she is distressed by the incident. Use a more tactful approach to invite the parents to meet with you to discuss the incident and their daughter's mental health and to allow you to answer any of their questions.

E5. _____ +3 This is appropriate. You are making it clear that her daughter is safe and that you want to involve the patient's parents in the treatment process.

E6. _____ −3 Unless the mother makes the specific request to speak with you directly, you should make a future appointment.

E7. _____ +5

DECISION POINT F

F1. _____ −3 Any substance use before the child's brain is fully developed, possibly around age 21–23, is also going to affect the child in ways that later use will not. It is okay to acknowledge that children and adolescents are naturally inquisitive and that some experiment with potentially harmful activities. This helps attenuate the child's shame or guilt and may help elicit more information. Continue to explore this topic as well as the patient's peer relationships.

F2. _____ −5 See F1. Additionally, the patient should be attending all of her milieu activities unless there is a good reason not to, but you would want to make that clear in a way that does not invoke more guilt for "failing" another authority figure. Moreover, it is inappropriate to "scold" the patient for anything.

F3. _____ +5

F4. _____ −2 Since the patient is a minor, you must involve her parents in the treatment process. However, in some states minors may confidentially receive treatment for substance use without parental consent.

F5. _____ +3 It would be a good idea to have the family involved in recovery. Again, if the state allows for the patient to receive confidential treatment without parental consent, then the patient must agree to family involvement.

DECISION POINT G

Depressed patients who exhibit difficulty concentrating can be misdiagnosed as having attention deficit hyperactivity disorder (ADHD). Match the following symptoms and signs with depression, ADHD, both, or neither. (Your score will be determined by the number of questions for which "both" is the correct answer.)

Symptom or Sign	Depression	ADHD	Both	Neither
G1. Often fails to give close attention to details or makes careless mistakes in schoolwork, work, or other activities		2		
G2. Often does not seem to listen when spoken to directly			2	
G3. Increase in goal-directed activity (either socially, at work or school, or sexually)				2
G4. Is often forgetful in daily activities			2	
G5. Insomnia or hypersomnia nearly every day	2			
G6. Markedly diminished interest or pleasure in all, or almost all, activities	2			
G7. Often loses things necessary for tasks or activities (e.g., toys, school assignments, pencils, books, or tools)			2	
G8. Psychomotor agitation			2	
G9. Inflated self-esteem or grandiosity				2
G10. Often has difficulty organizing tasks and activities			2	

YOUR TOTAL

Decision Point	Your Score	Ideal Best Score
A		7
B		22
C		5
D		16
E		12
F		8
G		10
Total		80

KEY CLINICAL POINTS

1. When assessing minors, the parents provide both a valuable source of history, consent for treatment of their child, and allies for follow-up care and compliance.
2. Experimentation with psychoactive substances is common in the adolescent age group. The psychiatrist should inquire about this at various times over the course of treatment.
3. A psychiatrist should be able to tactfully take a sexual history for this age group, especially prior to prescribing medications.
4. Regarding the ability of minors to consent to treatment, state laws vary based on factors including age, and type of treatment being delivered.

REFERENCES

American Psychiatric Association: Diagnostic and Statistical Manual of Mental Disorders, Fourth Edition, Text Revision. Washington DC, American Psychiatric Association, 2000

Hetrick SE, Merry SN, McKenzie J, Sindahl P, Proctor M. Selective serotonin reuptake inhibitors (SSRIs) for depressive disorders in children and adolescents. *Cochrane Database of Systematic Reviews* 2007, Issue 3.

McCarty CA, Weisz JR. Effects of psychotherapy for depression in children and adolescents: What we can (and can't) learn from meta-analysis and component profiling. J Am Acad Child Adolesc Psychiatry 2007;46:879–86

Sadock BJ, Sadock VA: Kaplan and Sadock's Synopsis of Psychiatry, 10th ed. Philadelphia, Lippincott Williams & Wilkins, 2007

Shea SC: The Practical Art of Suicide Assessment. Hoboken, NJ, Wiley, 2002

Weisz J R, McCarty C A, Valeri S M. Effects of psychotherapy for depression in children and adolescents: a meta-analysis. *Psychological Bulletin.* 2006;132(1):132–149

11

Child and Adolescent Psychiatry

What Do You Expect? My House Is Whacko

VIGNETTE PART 1

You are a child and adolescent psychiatrist working in an urban-setting group practice that includes adult psychiatrists. One of your colleagues refers Stacey, the 15-year-old daughter of one of his patients, for evaluation of what her father asserts is "the same problems I had when I was her age, but I never got help." The father understands from your conversation on the phone to arrange the appointment, that you wish to meet alone with Stacey for the first session. The father agreed to come in by himself for a second appointment. Stacey and her father show up for their evaluation appointment on time and immediately you note the constricted affect of the girl. Stacey does not offer you eye contact. She slowly enters the room, puts her feet on her chair, and rests her head against her knees. She is thin, wears glasses, and her hair is partially held from her face by a colorful, albeit dirty, headband with a silk flower affixed to one side. She is wearing a necklace of brightly colored jewelry, several bangles on her wrists, and her tennis shoes are decorated with flowers drawn in magic marker. She appears somewhat disheveled, is wearing sweatpants and a blue polo shirt with her school's emblem.

The father taps her head and says, loudly and assertively, "C'mon, Stace, get up. Don't behave like that in a doctor's office." He looks at you and shrugs.

You politely ask the father to step out of the office so you might interview Stacey alone. He agrees, but on his way out he uses his hand to lift the girl's head up and says to her, brusquely, "Come on, Stacey! Sit up! You are in a doctor's office. Is this how you behave?" The patient returns her head to her knees and the father leaves. You reintroduce yourself to the patient, and ask her how she is feeling right now. She does not answer. You wait. After a few minutes

you notice that her breathing has slowed and she appears to have fallen asleep. You move your chair closer and call her name. She moans quietly and shakes her head. You decide to shift the focus of your questions to something that might engage her, commenting on her colorful jewelry, how pretty it is, and ask whether she makes her own. She nods, although she does not lift her head. You ask what other hobbies she has. She does not answer and seems to have fallen asleep.

After a few moments you gently tap her on the shoulder and say that you know this may be uncomfortable for her to be in the psychiatrist's office, but you would like to know more about her. You ask her what time she went to sleep the previous night, a Sunday. She shrugs. You offer suggestions: "11 o'clock? 12 o'clock?" She holds up four fingers without moving her head from her knees. "Four in the morning?" She shrugs again. You ask what she was doing all night in her room until she fell asleep. Barely audible, she mumbles something about her computer. You ask her to please lift up her head because you want to hear what she has to say. After a couple of minutes she lifts her head, but pulls her long, somewhat unkempt hair over her eyes. She sighs loudly. "I don't want to be here,"she tells you in a soft, monotone voice. You wait. "It's not fair what they're doing to me," she says. "I can't help it if I can't sleep."

You ask if she stays up late every night. She says, using a tone suggesting some contempt, "What do you care?"You explain that you were asked to see if there is some way to help her with what seems to have become a difficult year. You then offer, "Sometimes kids stay up all night because it is quiet and they can think for themselves. Does this happen to you?" She nods. You ask, "What is it like for you at home?" Stacey pulls her hair aside, but looks off to the side. Her affect is still quite constricted, and there is little prosody in her speech. "My mother is always screaming at me to do my homework. So is my dad. I can't stand it." You comment that it must be difficult living in a home where everyone is always "on your case." She nods in agreement. "I do my work," she says, "although I do forget to turn in assignments, or I just lose them, or . . . I don't know. But the teachers are all idiots anyway. Why should I listen to them when they don't even know how to do the work they assign us?"

You ask if she has trouble staying organized. She nods. You say that she must be very smart to be able to accomplish so much in a very difficult school despite having trouble keeping track of things. She says, "Yeah, but they all know I'm smart. Some of the other kids are just idiots. I don't know how they got into my school." You ask if she likes her school. She says she does, but lately they have been picking on her "for some reason." You mention that you heard she sleeps through a lot of her classes. "Yeah," she says, "but I'm tired." You notice that there are only 10 minutes left to the session. You ask her to describe her mood. "Blah," she tells you. You ask if she feels depressed. "I don't know," she says, "probably." You ask if she has friends. She tells you she used to, but one friend did something to turn her other friends against her and now "everyone thinks I'm weird or something. I don't care. They're like little kids. They will not let go of things. Like picking my nose, or pretending I'm a cat. Well, they did let go of those things, but they haven't let go of saying that I lost my virginity to a dog. They've said that since first grade. I haven't lost my virginity."

A week later, the father comes alone for the individual appointment to which he had agreed. He thanks you for seeing Stacey and begins to list what he feels are the main concerns. "She was diagnosed with ADHD [attention deficit-hyperactivity disorder] when she was 10 and she took [methylphenidate] until last year. Her pediatrician prescribed it. She started complaining about headaches and was losing weight, so we stopped it last summer. She started out okay, but now it's impossible to get her out of bed in the morning. She usually misses her first class because I can't get her going. It is a daily struggle. Half the time she does not eat breakfast, even if I prepare something I know she likes. Then all the way to school she complains that her stomach hurts." He says she has not gained or lost any significant amount of weight. "She's always been thin, but she eats, usually in the evening or at night." "She stays up all night," continues the father, "playing alternate reality games on the computer. I've tried taking the computer out of her room, but she will start screaming and I have to give it back or all hell breaks loose."

The patient's father tells you he is also raising his son, Nick, 2 years older, who had a diagnosis of oppositional defiant disorder and ADHD, had started smoking marijuana, and was being treated at the same clinic by a different child and adolescent psychiatrist until recently when he refused to return for treatment. The father also has a young child with his current live-in girlfriend. Stacey and Nick's biological mother now lives a block away. "She's nuts." "I don't know what's wrong with her, but she is always screaming at Stacey." He explains that the situation at home was "unstable at best" for the past 10 years, since he and his wife separated and the mother of his youngest child moved into the first floor to live with him. Stacey's mother continued to live in the home on the second floor until a few months ago. "It's a duplex," he tells you, "but there is only one entrance; she had to come in through the first floor to get upstairs. There's no physical separation of the units."

Without prompting, the father tells you, "I've got depression. I've been taking an antidepressant for 10 years and it has helped a lot. I think I had the same attention problems as a kid as Stacey and Nick but I overcame them without medications. They really did not have much to treat it back then. I think they called me 'hyperactive' or something. It did not matter, though, because I had the brains." You ask what he does for a living. "I'm a biotech researcher here at the [Ivy League] University right up the street. But I do a lot of work at home from my computer." He is obese, wearing shorts and a wrinkled button-down, short-sleeved shirt.

Stacey is in eighth grade, attending a school for gifted children. He tells you that she has not had formal psychological testing except for a test in first grade, which indicated that she should be placed in a gifted academic program. ADHD was diagnosed by her pediatrician and the school psychologist when she was in second grade and a trial of long acting methylphenidate titrated to 36 mg daily, was initiated. This helped her focus; she did well in school and was considered one of the top students. She never had behavior problems. She has been at the same school since that time, and there are only 3 months remaining in the current year. The school is very demanding, and the students are required to maintain an 85% average to matriculate to each successive level. "Stacey is really smart. I mean *really* smart. She's also very artistic. Her teachers all love her." According to her father, during the past year she has been sleeping through classes and will crawl under a table in the classroom and sleep or surround her head with books at her desk. During a recent gym class she went to sleep in the corner on a mat, when the teacher asked her to get up and articipate in a game, she responded, "Why can't you just leave me alone?" Her behavior has been disruptive to each of her classes because she is "always sleeping," but when called upon to answer a question, she will lift up her head and know the right answer. Because of her "amazing intelligence" her behaviors have been overlooked until recently, when the school asked Stacey's father to have her evaluated by a psychiatrist. He tells you the school is considering expelling her unless she "shapes up" and "does what she's supposed to do. We had a meeting about this 2 weeks ago. I knew she was struggling a little bit for the past few months, but I had no idea they have been cutting her breaks all year."

He tells you, "We even went to the neurologist at the beginning of the year to see if she had narcolepsy or a sleep disorder." The results of a sleep study were negative, he tells you. The doctor at the sleep disorders clinic told the patient's father that her problem was due to "staying up all night."

DECISION POINT A

Given what you know about the patient so far, what steps would help you reach a clear diagnostic picture? Points awarded for correct and incorrect answers are scaled from best (+5) to unhelpful but not harmful (0) to dangerous (−5).

A1. _____ You know enough. ADHD had already been diagnosed and since she stopped taking long-acting methylphenidate 36 mg daily, her performance has suffered. As a result of the reemergence of her ADHD symptoms, she is having increasing difficulty in school, which you regard as the etiology of what seem to be mood symptoms.

A2. _____ You do not question the diagnosis of ADHD, but you believe that she has a mood disorder, probably depression, given her sleep disturbance, irritability, poor appetite, endorsement that she may be depressed, and her "blah" mood.

A3. _____ You do not question the diagnosis of ADHD, especially since her symptoms abated with the use of methylphenidate. There is also a strong family history of ADHD, both in her brother and possibly her father. You are concerned that she may have a mood disorder, so you request that the father bring the patient back the following week to continue the evaluation. You also provide a referral to obtain laboratory values for thyroid-stimulating hormone (TSH), a complete blood count (CBC) with differential, and urine drug toxicological analysis to rule out organic causes such as hypothyroidism, anemia, or drug abuse.

A4. _____ You suspect the diagnosis of ADHD may be appropriate, but you will require collateral information from teachers and more information from her father about how she behaves at home. You ask the father to fill out a Conner's ADHD metric and give him one for her primary teacher to fill out. You also request the father return with the patient the following week to further explore the possibility that she may have a mood disorder. You ask permission to speak with the mother for collateral history regarding that relationship and more family mental health history.

A5. _____ You require collateral information from the school and the parent about ADHD symptoms. You ask for permission to speak with the teacher, ask the father to fill out a Conner's ADHD metric, and give him one for her primary teacher to fill out. You ask for permission to speak with the mother for further collateral history, and you ask the father to

return the following week to obtain more detailed information about the patient's history, family life, social stressors, and any further symptoms that may suggest an additional diagnosis. You provide a referral to obtain laboratory values for TSH, a CBC with differential, and urine drug toxicological analysis to rule out organic causes such as hypothyroidism, anemia, or drug abuse.

VIGNETTE PART 2

The patient and her father return the following week to continue the evaluation. During the week you were able to speak with her primary teacher and school psychologist. They inform you that it is true that Stacey is "close to being asked not to return" the following year. They tell you her grades are good enough to finish the year, but not good enough to excuse her oppositional and disruptive behaviors. "She does things she knows she is not allowed to do," the teacher tells you. "Like having a cell phone in class, sleeping, or talking back. When we tell her about these things she acts oblivious, as though she never considered her actions to be against school policy. She knows the rules." The teacher did not fill out the Conner's metric, but she can tell you that Stacey has not been able to maintain concentration during the year. She knows the patient's mother stopped the ADHD medication and sees the negative effects of that discontinuation. "She is talented and smart, though," continues the teacher. "I feel bad. I know things in her home are not stable, but this is a unique school and the students have to maintain a high grade point average. Stacey is not able to do that this year. I ask her a question and it's like she's on another planet." She says that Stacey often forgets her homework, has left her bookbag and books at school on several occasions or forgets to bring them to school at all, and complains when she is asked to perform any sort of academic tasks in school. She tells you that her behavior seems oppositional this year and that she has never had a problem with hyperactivity. The school psychologist tells you that she meets regularly with Stacey, and the patient typically goes to sleep during their sessions. "Yes, it is annoying, but I let her sleep. I do paperwork while she sleeps in the chair."

You attempted three times during the week to reach the patient's mother. You left voice-mail messages asking her to please call you. You check with the patient's father and the number you have been trying is correct.

Stacey and her father are in the waiting room when you arrive at your office, and Stacey is asleep on a chair. You ask the patient to come into your office. After a great deal of effort by her father, the patient gets up, saunters into your office, plops down on a chair, and puts her feet on your desk. She is again somewhat disheveled, her sweatpants appear unwashed, and she presents similarly to the first visit. You ask her to please remove her feet from your desk and she refuses. "I'm tired," she tells you. You ask her again, and she reluctantly takes her feet down. Then she puts her feet on her chair as she had the first time you met. You ask her to please try and stay awake so you can learn more about her. "Why?" She demands. "Everyone is picking on me." She pounds her head with her fists. "I can't take this." You ask her what is bothering her right now. She looks at you incredulously for a moment, and then averts her gaze to your bookshelf. "You talked to my teacher. She told me. Now they're treating me like I'm retarded."

You assure her that you contacted her teacher to find out how she is doing in school because that is the area about which her family is most concerned. "I don't know," she tells you. "I'm sure I'm going to pass because I always do." Then she looks around the office. "How much time do we have left?" You ask her how late she stayed up the previous night. She shrugs. You offer that you know that sometimes kids will stay up late because it is quieter and they feel as though they can finally relax if there is too much commotion going on in the home during the day and evening. She says, "Yeah, I guess that is part of it. My mother is always screaming at me. She does not care about anything except my computer." You mention that you know her mother now lives out of the home. "I spend every stupid weekend with her. I can't stand it. All she does is cater to Nick. He's always doing stuff and never gets in trouble. I never do anything and I'm always in trouble. It's just not fair." You ask who Nick is and she responds, incredulously, "my brother. Didn't my father explain all of this to you?"

You ask if she ever becomes tearful and if she finds herself crying for no reason. She nods. You ask if she gets angry easily. She nods. Then she announces, "No, I've never tried to kill myself. I think that is stupid. My school counselor asks me that all the time." Then she sighs loudly and puts her head down on her knees. "People at my school are so stupid. They don't get me. They just want to punish me all the time. Now they think I'm crazy." You ask what she thinks. She does not respond. You mention that you notice that she seems angry today. Without lifting her head, she answers, "Well, I guess that is because maybe I hate it here?" You wait. "My mother was supposed to take me shopping. I waited for her to pick me up for FIVE HOURS!" She slams a fist against one of the arm rests, yet her affect seems unchanged, as if the reaction was entirely mechanical. "What was I supposed to do? I waited and waited, and then I got onto the computer. So, when she came home, guess what she did?" She looks off to the side. "She yelled at me. Big surprise." She shifts in her chair. "So, I refused to go to the store with her and she took Nick. She bought him stuff and then took him to dinner. I just sat at home. I called my dad to pick me up. The next day, she wanted me to come over and bake cookies. What the hell is that?" You note that despite the increased volume and occasional sarcastic tone, much of her speech is either devoid of affect, or with incongruent affect.

You inquire her how long she has felt like this. She tells you, "I don't know, for the past month. I guess since my mother moved out. I thought I would feel better because she wouldn't be there screaming at me every stupid second. I mean, it was

nice not having her yelling at me. I don't understand how my dad could bring this other woman to live in our home while he is still married to my mother. And they have a kid." You ask how long ago the other woman came to live with them. She says, "About 10 years ago. We have a duplex that is connected inside, so my mother lived upstairs and my father, Michael, and Nancy live downstairs." You ask where her bedroom is. "On the first floor, but it is full of boxes with my father's stuff in them. Nick lives in the basement. Sometimes I went upstairs and slept on my mother's couch."

You ask the patient if she has ever smoked cigarettes. She shakes her head "no." You ask about alcohol and she again shakes her head "no." When you ask about marijuana she does not reply. "Sometimes kids try smoking marijuana to see what it is like. Sometimes they smoke it every day or every week." Stacey remains still in her chair. "I'm not the police," you tell her. "I just need to know if you use marijuana or other drugs because it will help me better understand what's happening." She lifts her head and then looks around the room. "Are you going to tell my father?"

DECISION POINT B

The patient has indicated to you that she probably has tried marijuana and wants to know whether you will reveal this to her father. How should you respond? Points awarded for correct and incorrect answers are scaled from best (+5) to unhelpful but not harmful (0) to dangerous (−5).

B1. ____ "Yes." Explain to her that she is only 15 years old, and this is dangerous behavior for someone her age. Because she is a minor you are obligated to tell her father. Apologize for having to break her confidence, but it is for her own good.

B2. ____ "Yes." Explain that there are a several issues that you must share with her parents given her age. One is whether she is in danger of hurting herself or others, and the other is if she admits to using illicit drugs.

B3. ____ "No." Tell her that everything you share in the office is entirely confidential.

B4. ____ "No." Tell her that almost everything you share in the office is confidential except if you learn that she intends to harm or kill herself or others.

B5. ____ Ask her more questions about her usage. If she has tried it but no longer uses it, and if her drug toxicology screen results confirms this, you will keep this information confidential unless she again uses the drug.

B6. ____ Ask her more questions about her usage. If she is still using the drug with any frequency, you will have to share this information with her father as this would represent a dangerous behavior about which her parents must be made aware.

B7. ____ Ask her more questions about her usage. If she used it in the past, has stopped, and can agree to be honest about her use with you and even submit to unannounced urine toxicology screening (if this is permitted by your state law), you will keep her confidence for now. Discuss with her the evidence that most people with substance abuse problems have a greater chance of maintaining abstinence if their family is involved.

VIGNETTE PART 3

You thank Stacey for being honest with you and sharing details that are obviously troubling. "Well, what do you expect?" She asks. "My house is wacko." You ask if she ever did anything to harm herself. "I cut," she says plainly. She lifts up her head and holds out her right arm. You note several superficial horizontal cuts near her wrist. You ask if she ever tried to kill herself by cutting. "No." she responds. "I told you I don't want to kill myself. Don't you listen?" You tell her, "Sometimes kids cut themselves because it makes them feel better. Sometimes it is because of the pain, seeing the blood, or both. When do you cut yourself?" She shrugs. Then she offers, "When I'm angry. I also get headaches. Like right now." You ask if she ever took pills for her headaches. She answers, "Yes." You ask if she ever took more than 2 tablets for a really bad headache. "Yes," she tells you. "Once I took about 8 or 10 and I went to sleep. I ended up waking up and puking." You ask if she intended to die. "No. I told you that already. Don't you listen?" She admits she took the pills after a fight with her mother about a year ago. Since then she admits only to cutting, which she says she last did a few days earlier after an argument with her father about schoolwork.

She tells you she does not have racing thoughts. "They ask me this at school sometimes when I act goofy." She tells you she often ruminates about things, but was never told by anyone that she spoke too fast or that her speech was unintelligible. She denies having any sexual partners and never goes on spending sprees ("I save my money"). You ask about a decreased need for sleep, which she denies.

You ask her what she likes to do. "Nothing," she tells you. You mention that you heard that she is a talented artist. "Yeah," she says. "I'm good." You ask what her favorite media is. "Drawing and painting," she replies, dryly. You wait. "I haven't been doing it much, lately." You ask why. "I just don't feel like it. I don't feel like doing anything. Just the computer, and that just gets me into trouble so I don't know why I even bother trying to use it." You recall she said she lost a lot of friends. You ask if there is anyone with whom she still does things. "My brother," she says. "We hang out in the basement sometimes. I don't like his friends very much, though. They're jerks and they pick on me." You ask how long she has not felt like doing the things she normally enjoys. She thinks for a while then responds, "I don't know. Maybe a year. Maybe more. Maybe less."

You ask her what her biggest worries are. She puts her head back down and shifts in her chair. "I guess school," she tells you. "Or maybe they're going to send me off someplace to get rid of me." She wipes her eyes on her sweatpants and then lets out a wail that begins softly and then picks up volume. You wait. You note that she does not seem to be crying. She stops suddenly. "Can I go now?" As the session is over, you agree.

DECISION POINT C

Given what you know about this patient, what is your differential diagnosis? +2 points are given for correct answers, and −2 points for incorrect answers.

AXIS I:	
AXIS II:	

DECISION POINT D

In adolescent females, a diagnosis of ADHD has been shown in several studies to be a significant risk factor for which of the following (+2 points are given for correct answers and −2 points for incorrect answers):

D1. _____ Long-term psychosocial impairment
D2. _____ Suicide
D3. _____ Psychiatric hospitalization
D4. _____ Chronic course
D5. _____ Major depression
D6. _____ Mania

D7. _____ Oppositional defiant disorder
D8. _____ Conduct disorder
D9. _____ Illicit drug use/abuse
D10. _____ Anxiety disorders

DECISION POINT E

If you conclude that comorbid ADHD, major depressive disorder, and cannabis abuse can be diagnosed in this patient, what would be the best approach to treatment, from both psychopharmacological and psychotherapeutic modalities? Points awarded for correct and incorrect answers are scaled from best (+5) to unhelpful but not harmful (0) to dangerous (−5).

E1. _____ Treat the substance abuse first, then the major depressive disorder, and then the ADHD.
E2. _____ Treat the major depressive disorder first. This will probably reveal that the patient has been using marijuana to self-medicate and should have an easier time abstaining from its use. Use fluoxetine, the best studied selective serotonin reuptake inhibitor (SSRI) for adolescents, to treat the major depressive disorder. The ADHD will probably resolve as it was most likely the result of being "stoned" all the time and therefore leaving the patient unable to concentrate and suffering from amotivational syndrome.
E3. _____ Treat the ADHD first. Her subsequent demoralization and difficulties in school most likely were the etiology of the major depressive disorder and the substance abuse. If she continues to have symptoms once the ADHD is controlled, then treat the major depressive disorder and substance abuse concurrently.
E4. _____ Use the regular formulation of methylphenidate or amphetamine to treat the ADHD as this is the most likely therapy to help the patient's ADHD symptoms. It will also lift her mood as she will have more energy and not feel the need to self-medicate with marijuana.
E5. _____ Once the substance abuse has been treated, begin with either long-acting methylphenidate or amphetamine as these are not easily abused. Alternatively begin with bupropion which, although considered a third-line treatment for ADHD, will also help with depressive symptoms.

ANSWERS: SCORING, RELATIVE WEIGHTS, AND COMMENTS

DECISION POINT A

A1. _____ −5 Although the diagnosis of ADHD may be correct, this patient has symptoms that sug-

gest a variety of other diagnoses (see Decision Point C). The patient's story is complicated, and she is only mildly cooperative during the interview. Because of their patients' developmental age and minor status, child and adolescent psychiatrists must make every effort to gather collateral information in addition to further exploration of the patient's psychiatric, developmental, academic, familial, medical, social, and personal histories. This would not be good practice with an adult who presented in such a fashion.

A2. _____ −3 Although the diagnosis of ADHD may be correct and your thoughts about a presumptive diagnosis of depression may represent a greater perspective than that suggested by answer A1, the mood symptoms may be related to other factors. In addition, because of their patients' developmental age and minor status, child and adolescent psychiatrists must also make every effort to gather collateral information in addition to further exploration of the patient's psychiatric, developmental, academic, familial, medical, social, and personal histories.

A3. _____ +3 Although you are not skeptical about the diagnosis of ADHD given the prior diagnosis at age 10, her positive response to ADHD medication, and a strong likelihood of familial genetic loading for ADHD, this answer suggests that your thinking has some basis in evidence. Numerous studies are highly suggestive of a heritable component to ADHD. However, ADHD is a clinical diagnosis, and it is not wise to base a diagnosis upon response to a specific treatment. You do note the possibility of a substance abuse issue by asking for a urine toxicology screen, and you are searching for any possible medical reasons for her symptoms. You have not made up your mind about other possible diagnoses, and ask the father to return for further evaluation. However, it is imperative to get collaborative reports of the patient's behaviors and symptoms from other stakeholders given the poor co-operation of the patient and only the father's perspective on a family situation that is clearly chaotic and may be, at the very least, exacerbating her symptoms, especially because she mentions her own anger concerning her father's decision to invite his girlfriend to live in the family home while the biological mother lived upstairs.

A4. _____ +3 By being skeptical about the prior diagnosis of ADHD, considering a mood disorder, and seeking to further verify these diagnoses by obtaining collateral information from parents and teachers, including the use of metrics, your evaluation is proceeding in a more appropriate and effective manner. However, this answer does not include other important aspects of a full diagnostic evaluation, such as the patient's psychiatric, developmental, academic, familial, medical, social, and personal histories.

A5. _____ +5 You remain skeptical about all diagnoses and make efforts to obtain further information, both from the patient, her father, and other stakeholders. You also ask for metrics to help assess the overall picture and create a baseline measurement to which you can later compare results once treatment is initiated. Finally, you attempt to rule out medical causes of her symptoms as well as laboratory proof of substance abuse. This is the most thorough of the choices offered.

DECISION POINT B

Generally, studies have repeatedly demonstrated that the greatest likelihood of success for the individual patient in the treatment of substance abuse disorders is seen when family and peers are involved. Of concern, of course, is maintaining the therapeutic alliance with the patient so that there is trust and open communication between patient and doctor. In this particular patient, you have not yet determined whether there is a significant substance abuse problem. As a result, clinicians are divided regarding whether to share this sensitive information immediately with the patient's caregivers or to wait until it is determined whether the substance abuse is significant enough to warrant specific treatment. Many worry that if the therapeutic alliance is broken so easily and quickly before the substance abuse issue is substantiated, any treatment will be compromised, whether it is for the alleged substance abuse, major depressive disorder, ADHD, or other diagnoses. On the other hand, it can be argued that "nipping it in the bud" by addressing the potential for substance abuse with involvement of the family immediately will yield a greater degree of patient safety, as well as treatment of the comorbidities.

Regarding drug-testing of minors, laws can differ from state to state. For the past 50 years, laws have been changed to allow for minors to obtain treatment without parental consent for specific concerns such as sexually transmitted diseases, alcohol and substance abuse treatment, mental health care, and contraception. The clinician should clarify the limits of these rights as some states mandate reporting, whereas others prohibit it. Some states allow for treatment of alcohol-related disorders while insisting on parental consent for other substances.

B1. _____ −1 As stated above, many clinicians will feel obligated to involve the family from the start, even if the substance abuse has not been substantiated, because of the risks involved. However, given that you just met this patient, it would be wise to establish a better rapport with the patient to pave the way for her acceptance of your "need" to break this confidence.

B2. _____ −1 For the same reasons as stated in answer B1, if you wish to involve the patient's family immediately, the rapport described in the vignette thus far is not sufficient given the unsubstantiated and unexplored diagnosis of actual substance abuse.

B3. _____ −5 This is not true. Although most information shared in the doctor-patient relationship may not be disclosed, specific concerns are not considered confidential. For example, if the patient admits to engaging in dangerous behaviors, threatening suicide or homicide, she is a minor, and her parents should be informed. If she is threatening homicide, you have a "duty to protect" the intended victim according to the Tarasoff ruling.

B4. _____ +3 Although this is true, because she is a minor, dangerous behaviors should be shared with her parents to help with treatment. This point should be explained in a way that does not prompt the patient to deliberately withhold information for fear of parental or legal reprisals. As stated in the first two answers in Decision Point B, the establishment of a strong therapeutic alliance and solid rapport will aide in delivering this information without compromising the patient's likelihood of sharing sensitive material.

B5. _____ +3 Given that you do not yet know the extent of her substance abuse, further exploration of her use of illicit substances will help you develop a clearer clinical picture and give the 15-year-old patient incentive to maintain abstinence before you share the information with her parents. This approach may prove therapeutic and allow for the clinician to maintain the alliance should the patient prove unable to maintain abstinence per their agreement In some parts of the country, especially in California, there is a movement toward a harm reduction approach, in which the clinician meets the patient where he or she is in terms of the abuse and uses motivational interviewing techniques to help him or her see the substance abuse as a problem.

B6. _____ +1 Further evaluation of the substance use will determine the severity of the problem. If the patient's abuse of substances is significant, this constitutes risky and dangerous behavior. It is then up to the clinician to decide whether to break confidence and involve the family or to allow the patient to volunteer for treatment. Two important caveats are as follows. The particular state that the patient lives in may allow for her to seek treatment for substance abuse without prior parental consent, so breaking this confidence could undermine any further treatment for her possible comorbid diagnoses. Depending on the patient's domestic situation, involvement of the family in the treatment of substance abuse has been demonstrated to be more effective than allowing the patient to manage this problem on her own.

B7. _____ +5 This answer allows the patient to feel as though she is collaborating with you to maintain sobriety. The approach is amenable to further development of a solid rapport and therapeutic relationship but leaves open the possibility that her parents may become involved specifically in the issue of her substance abuse if she is unable to address the problem on her own. It also includes useful psycho-education about the potential benefits of involving her family in this treatment. Your discussions with her school faculty have been focused on her behavior and academic performance.

DECISION POINT C

Axis I:	(+2) Attention Deficit-Hyperactivity Disorder, Inattentive Type; (−2) Attention Deficit-Hyperactivity Disorder, Combined Type; (+2) Depressive Disorder, Not Otherwise Specified; (+2) Dysthymic Disorder; (+2) Oppositional Defiant Disorder; (−2) Conduct Disorder; (−2) Rule out Cannabis Abuse; (+2) Rule out Substance-Induced Mood Disorder; (+2) Rule out Bipolar Disorder; (−2) Major Depressive Disorder; (−2) Rule out Anxiety Disorder, Not Otherwise Specified; (−2) Adjustment Disorder
Axis II:	(−2) Strong Cluster B Traits; (−2) Borderline Personality Disorder; (−2) Narcissistic Personality Disorder; (−2) Histrionic Personality Disorder; (−2) Schizoid Personality Disorder; (−2) Borderline Personality Disorder

Attention Deficit-Hyperactivity Disorder, Inattentive Type (+2). This patient is disorganized, is unable to sustain attention, does not seem to listen when spoken to directly, is not completing her academic work, often either leaves her book bag at home or forgets to take it home from school, refuses to participate in academic activities that require attention, seems internally preoccupied, and is often forgetful in daily activity. She subsequently meets the criteria for the inattentive aspect of ADHD at school, and her father's reports suggest similar impairments at home.

Attention Deficit-Hyperactivity Disorder, Combined Type (−2). She does not meet criteria for hyperactivity or impulsivity. Her disruptive behaviors are more likely explained by oppositional defiant disorder.

Depressive Disorder, Not Otherwise Specified (+2). The patient endorses anhedonia, sleep disturbance, difficulty with concentration, and irritability. Subsequently, at this early stage in your evaluation, she does not meet the criteria for a major depressive disorder or episode. Some of her answers are ambivalent, leaving open the question of whether she has a dysthymic disorder or suffered a major

depressive episode 1 year ago when she ingested 8–10 headache tablets. Further evaluation may help establish one or both of these diagnoses.

Dysthymic Disorder (+2). As stated in the explanation for Depressive D/O, NOS, further evaluation of the patient's symptoms and time course will help determine whether she meets criteria for a Dysthymic D/O. She may have had a Major Depressive Episode on top of a preexisting Dysthymia, when considering her intentional ingestion of Tylenol one year ago. For children and adolescents, the criteria requires symptoms lasting at least one year, instead of the two years required for this diagnosis in adults.

Oppositional Defiant Disorder (+2). Information from teacher and school psychologist, reports from her father, and her behavior in your office all suggest a pattern of negativistic, hostile, and defiant behavior lasting at least 6 months, during which she often loses her temper, argues with adults, refuses to comply with adults' requests or rules, blames others for her mistakes or misbehavior, is easily annoyed by others, seems irritable, and is angry and resentful. These behaviors have caused her to be close to expulsion by her school despite her ability to perform academically, and it is not apparent that these criteria were met specifically during a mood disorder.

Conduct Disorder (−2). This patient does not meet the criteria for conduct disorder, which requires three or more of the following criteria in the past 12 month with at least 1 criterion present in the past 6 months: aggression to people and animals; destruction of property; deceitfulness or theft; or serious violations of rules.

Rule out Cannabis Abuse (−2). The patient has intimated that she may have used marijuana by asking if you intend to tell her father. She has not admitted to using marijuana and you do not have results of a urine toxicology screen. Both ADHD and depression both have strong links to comorbid substance abuse, so this issue requires further evaluation.

Rule out Substance-Induced Mood Disorder (+2). Until you have established the severity of the patient's cannabis use, you must entertain the possibility that her current symptoms are subsequent to this use. This patient certainly has severe psychosocial stressors, including the possibility of her expulsion from school, interpersonal conflicts with family members, loss of friendships, and a chaotic home environment. However, given the limited history you have obtained thus far, it is difficult to determine how resilient this patient may be to the psychosocial stressors versus the effects of a possible substance abuse problem. Determining this will affect your treatment strategy.

Rule out Bipolar Disorder (+2). This patient exhibits an irritable mood and mild grandiosity, belittling her classmates and teachers as not being as intelligent as she is. However, her self-esteem does not appear to be overly inflated, especially as she is known to be intelligent and talented and since the first grade been in gifted academic programs. She does not describe a decreased need for sleep, but a reversal of her days and nights. She easily falls asleep in your office, the waiting room, and in school. The cardinal symptoms of pediatric mania, as described by researchers, including Robins, Guze, and Staton et al., in an attempt to differentiate true mania from ADHD by looking past the more nonspecific symptom of irritability, focus more on extreme forms of grandiosity, elation, and racing thoughts. This patient does not describe racing thoughts, nor does she describe any of the other bipolar disorder-specific symptoms. She is easily distracted, but her symptoms seem more related to ADHD and depressive symptoms. However, a link between ADHD as a risk factor for mania has been suggested by several researchers so ruling this out by taking further history, especially from collateral informants, is important. If you do determine she has mood bipolarity, this will affect your choice of pharmacotherapy.

Major Depressive Disorder (−2). Given the ambivalence of the patient's description of her mood, the reference to an intentional ingestion of 8–10 headache tablets in the context of a fight with her mother, and your suspicion that she has at least four of the five criteria currently for a major depressive disorder, you may find she qualifies for major depressive episode, severe without psychotic features, in full remission. Currently, however, she does not meet the criteria as explained above under depressive disorder, not otherwise specified.

Rule out Anxiety Disorder, Not Otherwise Specified (−2). Although a link between ADHD and anxiety disorders has been demonstrated in the literature, this patient does not describe nor exhibit symptoms of panic disorder, social phobia, obsessive-compulsive disorder, posttraumatic stress disorder, acute stress disorder, or generalized anxiety disorder. Unless you uncover symptoms of any of these anxiety disorders during further evaluation, at this point in she does not qualify even for a rule-out diagnosis.

Adjustment Disorder (−2). To meet the criteria for an adjustment disorder, this patient must have developed her symptoms within 3 months of the onset of a stressor. According to the patient's father, she learned only in the past 2 weeks of the possibility of her expulsion from school. Other psychosocial stressors that have been described by both the father and the patient have been ongoing.

Strong Cluster B Traits (−2). The difference between "traits" and a "disorder" typically implies an enduring character-logic pattern that causes clinically significant distress or impairment in social, occupational, or other important areas of functioning. Diagnosing a personality disorder in an adolescent or child is fraught with controversy and can cause irreparable damage to the patient by virtue of labeling, both from the patient's personal experience and by the preconceived notions of others including clinicians. According to the DSM-IV-TR's strict criteria, personality disorder categories may be applied to children or adolescents in those relatively unusual instances in which the individuals particular maladaptive personality traits appear to be pervasive, persistent, and unlikely to be limited to a particular axis I illness. To diagnose a personality disorder in an individual under age 18, the features must have been present for at least one year. All people have personalities, and many have specific traits that can be understood as the individual's adaptive or maladaptive behavioral patterns. This patient exhibits some traits that are nonspecific but tied to a personality disorder, such as impulsivity and irritability in antisocial personality disorder. However, she clearly does not meet the criteria for this much more serious disorder, which is the one personality disorder that cannot be diagnosed until age 18.

Subsequently:

Rule out Borderline Personality Disorder (−2). She describes losing her friends or being picked on, which may suggest a pattern of unstable interpersonal relationships. She continues to engage in self-injurious behavior, namely cutting. Her affect during your interviews features a rapid movement from what seems like an isolation of affect to marked reactivity, suggestive of borderline personality disorder, although these mood shifts are very transient, not meeting the criterion of lasting a few hours to a few days.

Additionally, this patient's maladaptive coping strategies may be more temporary, related primarily to Axis I diagnoses plus living in a dysfunctional family environmental and being part of a highly demanding academic setting. According to strict DSM-IV-TR criteria, it is considered premature to ascribe personality disorders to adolescents as their personalities or character structures are still undergoing major, dynamic evolution.

Rule out Histrionic Personality Disorder (−2). She dresses in an inimical style that she may use to attract attention to herself, suggesting a histrionic personality disorder; however, she is also known to be artistic, and the style is not considered provocative or sexually seductive.

Rule-Out Narcissistic Personality Disorder (−2). Her admissions that she is smart and talented, more so than her peers or teachers, that no one understands her, and that she may behave as she likes despite the rules of the school suggesting a sense of entitlement, plus her arrogant, haughty behaviors indicate a narcissistic personality disorder. However these behaviors and attitudes may also be at least partially explained by oppositional defiant disorder at this stage in her development. Therefore, although it may be true this patient is developing the maladaptive aspects of a narcissistic personality structure, it is too early to make such a diagnosis or even a rule out.

Rule out Schizoid Personality Disorder (−2). She has not described any sexual interests, but you have not explored this area yet. She does not have friends but has had friends in the past. If she felt better, it is likely that she would wish for more social interaction. She chooses solitary activities, but this choice is better described by depressive symptoms than by a personality disorder. Finally, although she admits to being anhedonic, this is not the same as the criterion of taking pleasure in few, if any, activities associated with schizoid personality disorder.

DECISION POINT D

D1. ____ +2 Long-term psychosocial impairment. Studies have demonstrated an increased occurrence of impaired functioning in work, social, and family life.

D2. ____ +2 Suicide. Clinical outcomes of patients with adolescent-onset major depressive disorder into adulthood compared with control subjects without psychiatric illness include a high rate of suicide (7.7%), a fivefold increased risk for first suicide attempt, and a twofold increased risk of major depressive disorder.

D3. ____ +2 Psychiatric hospitalization. Studies have demonstrated an increased occurrence of psychiatric and medical hospitalization.

D4. ____ +2 Chronic course. Given the high risk of comorbidity between ADHD and major depressive disorder and the significant impairments associated with each individual disorder, the severity of the major depressive disorder in the context of ADHD has a higher likelihood of ongoing morbidity and disability, as well as poor long-term prognosis.

D5. ____ +2 Major depression. Recent studies have demonstrated a range of a 2- to 5.1-fold increase in the development of major depressive disorder compared with that for control subjects, after controlling for comorbid conditions. This finding is considered to be of greater significance in adolescent than in adult females. The major depressive disorder was found to be more severe, causing greater impairment and increased suicidality.

D6. ____ +2 Mania. Several new studies have documented robust associations between ADHD, bipolar disorder, and conduct disorder in this population.

D7. ____ +2 Oppositional defiant disorder. Continuity from one diagnosis to another (heterotypic) has been shown to be significant from depression to anxiety and anxiety to depression, from ADHD to oppositional defiant disorder, and from anxiety and conduct disorder to substance abuse. Girls are overrepresented in the heterotypic subset compared with boys.

D8. ____ +2 Conduct disorder. ADHD in adolescent females has been associated with significant increase in risk for conduct disorder, independent of major depressive disorder.

D9. ____ +2 Illicit drug use/abuse. Adolescents with major depressive disorder and untreated ADHD have been shown by several studies to have a greater risk of developing substance abuse disorders and, more significantly, alcohol-related disorders. However, it should be noted that one new study (Bieder-man, et al) demonstrated that there is no evidence of psychostimulant treatment for ADHD having a protective effect against the development of substance abuse disorders into adulthood. Subsequently, more studies are warranted, especially those that examine female youth, before we conclude there is no protective effect.

D10. ____ +2 Anxiety disorders. Newer studies have demonstrated a significant association between major depressive disorder and increased risk for anxiety disorders. Continuity from one diagnosis to another (heterotypic) has been shown to be significant from depression to anxiety and anxiety to depression, from ADHD to oppositional defiant disorder, and from anxiety and conduct disorder to substance abuse. Girls are overrepresented in the heterotypic subset compared with boys.

DECISION POINT E

In general, before you can begin treating the ADHD or the major depressive disorder, you must first determine the severity of this patient's use or abuse of cannabis. You also need to further explore the magnitude and extent of the patient's mood symptoms and reevaluate the patient's diagnosis of ADHD. Given that there are multiple layers of pathological conditions in this patient, including a presumptive diagnosis of ADHD, it is necessary to further evaluate possible risky behaviors or abuse of other substances. Although the patient presents with some neurovegetative symptoms of depression such as anhedonia, sleep disturbance, appetite disturbance, and irritability (specific symptoms for depression in children and adolescents), these symptoms may also be explained by the abuse of marijuana or the diagnosis of ADHD. Address the abuse of marijuana using motivational interviewing (MI), cognitive behavioral therapy, and, if possible, family therapy (FT). MI has been shown to be very effective in helping patients overcome any ambivalence they may have about their substance use and is used to help foment a determination by patients to overcome the abuse or addiction. CBT, especially in combination with SSRIs has been shown to have the most significant impact upon more severe forms of, depression if added after the SSRI is initiated during the acute phase. Patients were less able to benefit from psychotherapy while suffering from the worst of the depressive symptoms.

FT is typically underused in treatments because of difficulties in initiating such treatment with families and ongoing compliance if treatment has started or because the family itself is so fragmented and/or chaotic that bringing members in for treatment of the "identified patient" seems impossible. However, it has been demonstrated that a child's presentation is heavily influenced by environmental factors, specifically those within the family. From a diagnostic perspective, simply having the opportunity to explore the variety of family factors, including parental styles, patterns of interaction, and family dynamics, through direct observation will yield a more comprehensive and valuable understanding of the etiology of the child's presentation. Moreover, the opportunity to help the family reorganize what may be (and in the case of this child is) a maladaptive and dysfunctional multipersonal system that is focused on the individual patient will enable the family to reduce as much as possible the variety of individual systems whose function worsens the individual patient's psychopathology and reinforces negative and impaired familial function. In other words, helping the child to overcome his or her illness is of limited utility if he or she returns to the toxic environment that helped create or exacerbate it. In this particular case, family therapy could prove to be immensely challenging but possibly have the greatest impact if the family agrees to enter into this therapy.

If one wishes to initiate treatment of the ADHD, use of a long-acting stimulant formulation of methylphenidate, which cannot be abused owing to its unique pill construction, or the extended release formulations of amphetamine or methylphenidate, which have a lower potential likelihood of abuse, is recommended. Alternatively, if the patient does not have a seizure disorder, a history of clinically significant head trauma, or an eating disorder, a trial of bupropion because it treats the ADHD as well as depressive symptoms or atomoxetine because of its low potential for abuse may be useful.

Subsequently, numerous options are possible, including approaching each problem simultaneously. It is often difficult to sequence treatments in patients such as this one. In this particular patient, because we are still missing a lot of significant information that will influence treatment, we can attempt to parse out our approach according to what we do know, as follows:

E1. ____ +3 Treat the substance abuse first, then the major depressive disorder, and then the ADHD.

E2. ____ +3 Although sobriety may not be a useful endpoint, the patient's substance abuse is probably contributing to her mood symptoms. If the mood symptoms did not precede the substance abuse and in this patient this is unlikely, initiation of fluoxetine, the best studied SSRI for adolescents to treat the major depressive disorder is a good first step. Concurrent treatment of the ADHD while a patient is actively abusing marijuana has been demonstrated to have little impact on either the addiction or the ADHD unless the addiction is addressed first. Once the substance use has been addressed, rapid commencement of treatment of the ADHD is more effective. Whether the ADHD will probably resolve as it was most likely the result of being "stoned" all the time and therefore leaving the patient unable to concentrate and suffering from amotivational syndrome is a questionable assumption.

E3. ____ +3 If the ADHD is shown to be the cause of demoralization, academic failure, or other reasons for "self-medication," concurrent treatment of both the substance abuse and the ADHD may be most effective. Use of pharmacological agents without strong abuse potential for the treatment of ADHD, such as bupropion (assuming no history of significant head trauma or seizure disorder) or atomoxetine, is typically well tolerated, even in the context of abuse of marijuana. Bupropion has been demonstrated to be effective in the treatment of ADHD in adolescents with ADHD and depression or mood disorders and substance abuse. Another more recent pharmacological intervention is the use of modafinil, although the literature on the use of this agent is lacking.

E4. _____ −5 The regular formulations of psychostimulants, including methylphenidate and amphetamine, are easily and commonly crushed, snorted, or otherwise ingested with the intention of substance abuse. In a patient with a substance abuse disorder, this will only contribute to the problem.

E5. _____ +3 For the same reasons as described above, these treatments are acceptable.

YOUR TOTAL

Decision Point	Score	Ideal Score
A		11
B		12
C		12
D		20
E		12
Total		67

KEY CLINICAL POINTS

1. Children and adolescents often present with symptoms that overlap several diagnoses. Before reaching a diagnosis, careful evaluation of reports by collateral informants, including caregivers, teachers, and any stakeholders is imperative.

2. As with all patients, the strength of the therapeutic relationship will inform the willingness of a child or adolescent to share sensitive information.

3. The child or adolescent must be made aware that potentially lethal information may be shared with the patient's caregivers, such as suicidal ideation, homicidal ideation, or drug abuse.

REFERENCES

American Academy of Pediatrics: AAFP Statement of Policy on Adolescent Health Care: American Academy of Family Physicians Web site. http://www.aafp.org/online/en/home/policy/policies/s/substanceabuse.html

Angold A, Costello EJ: Depressive co-morbidity in children and adolescents: empirical, theoretical and methodological issues. Am J Psychiatry 1993; 150:1779–1791

Angold A, Costello J, Erkanli A: Co-morbidity. J Child Psychol Psychiatry 1999;40:57–87

Biederman J, Monuteaux MC, Spencer T, Wilens TE, Macpherson HA, Faraone SV: Stimulant therapy and risk for subsequent substance use disorders in male adults with ADHD: a naturalistic controlled 10-year follow-up study. Am J Psychiatry. 2008 May;165(5):597–603

Biederman J, Ball SW, Monuteaux MC, Mick E, Spencer TJ, McCreary M, Cote M, Faraone SV: New insights into the co-morbidity between ADHD and major depression in adolescent and young adult females. J Am Acad Child Adolesc Psychiatry 2008; 467:427–434

Biederman J, Faraone SV, Mick E, Spencer T, Wilens T, Kiely K, Guite J, Ablon JS, Reed E, Warburton R.: High risk for attention deficit hyperactivity disorder among children of parents with childhood onset of the disorder: a pilot study. Am J Psychiatry 1995; 152:431–435

Biederman J, Faraone S, Mick E, Wozniak J, Chen L, Ouellette C, Marrs A, Moore P, Garcia J, Mennin D, Lelon E: Attention-deficit hyperactivity disorder and juvenile mania: an overlooked co-morbidity? J Am Acad Child Adolesc Psychiatry 1996; 35:997–1008

Biederman J, Faraone SV, Wozniak J, Montuteaux MC: Parsing the association between bipolar, conduct, and substance use disorders: a familial risk analysis. Biol Psychiatry 2000; 48:1037–1044

Biederman J, Mick E: Wozniak J, Monuteaux M, Galdo M, Farone S. Can a subtype of conduct disorder linked to bipolar disorder be identified? Integration of findings from the Massachusetts General Hospital Pediatric Psychopharmacology Research Program. Biol Psychiatry 2003; 53:952–960

Biederman J, Newcorn J, Sprich S: Co-morbidity of attention deficit hyperactivity disorder with conduct, depressive, anxiety, and other disorders. Am J Psychiatry 1991; 148:564–577

Biederman J, Monuteaux MC, Mick E, Spencer T, Wilens TE, Klein KL, Price JE, Faraone SV: Psychopathology in females with attention-deficit/hyperactivity disorder: a controlled, five-year prospective study. Biol Psychiatry 2006; 60:1098–1105

Biederman J, Petty CR, Wilens TE, Fraire MG, Purcell CA, Mick E, Monuteaux MC, Faraone SV: Familial risk analyses of attention deficit hyperactivity disorder and substance use disorders. Am J Psychiatry 2008; 165:107– 115

Birmaher B, Ryan ND, Williamson DE, Brent DA, Kaufman J, Dahl RE, Perel J, Nelson B: Childhood and adolescent depression: a review of the past 10 years. Part I. J Am Acad Child Adolesc Psychiatry. 1996; 35:1427–1439

Carlisle J, Shickle D, Cork M, McDonagh A: Concerns over confidentiality may deter adolescents from consulting their doctors: a qualitative exploration. J Med Ethics 2006; 32:133–137

Costello EJ, Mustillo S, Erkanli A, Keeler G, Angold A: Prevalence and development of psychiatric disorders in childhood and adolescence. Arch Gen Psychiatry 2003; 60:837–844

Curry J, Rohde P, Simons A, Silva S, Vitiello B, Kratochvil C, Reinecke M, Feeny N, Wells K, Pathak S, Weller E, Rosenberg D, Kennard B, Robins M, Ginsburg G, March J, TADS Team: Predictors and moderators of acute outcome in the Treatment for Adolescents with Depression Study (TADS). J Am Acad Child Adolesc Psychiatry 2006; 45:1427–1439

Daviss WB, Bentivoglio P, Racusin R, Brown KM, Bostic JQ, Wiley L: Bupropion SR in adolescents with combined attention-deficit/hyperactivity disorder and depression. J Am Acad Child Adolesc Psychiatry 2001; 40:307–314

Faraone SV, Biederman J, Mick E, Williamson S, Wilens T, Spencer T, Weber W, Jetton J, Kraus I, Pert J, Zallen B: Family study of girls with attention deficit hyperactivity disorder. Am J Psychiatry 2000; 157:1077–1083

Faraone SV, Doyle AE: Genetic influences on attention deficit hyperactivity disorder. Curr Psychiatry Rep 2000; 2:143–146

Galanter CA, Leibenluft E: Frontiers between attention deficit hyperactivity disorder and bipolar disorder. Child Adolesc Psychiatr Clin N Am. 2008; 17:325–346, viii–ix

Garner BR, Godley SH, Funk RR: Predictors of early therapeutic alliance among adolescents in substance abuse treatment. J Psychoactive Drugs 2008; 40:55–65

Goodman R, Stevenson J: A twin study of hyperactivity, II: the aetiological role of genes, family relationships and perinatal adversity. J Child Psychol Psychiatry 1989; 30:691–709

Greene RW, Biederman J, Faraone SV, Monuteaux MC, Mick E, DuPre EP, Fine CS, Goring JC: Social impairment in girls with ADHD: patterns, gender comparisons, and correlates. J Am Acad Child Adolesc Psychiatry 2001; 40:704–710

Griswold KS, Aronoff H, Kernan JB, Kahn LS: Adolescent substance use and abuse: recognition and management. Am Fam Physician 2008; 77:331– 336

Hechtman L: Genetic and neurobiological aspects of attention deficit hyperactive disorder: a review. J Psychiatry Neurosci 1994; 19:193–201

Hurtig T, Ebeling H, Taanila A, Miettunen J, Smalley SL, McGough JJ, Loo SK, Järvelin MR, Moilanen IK: ADHD symptoms and subtypes: relationship between childhood and adolescent symptoms. J Am Acad Child Adolesc Psychiatry 2007; 46:1605–1613

Josephson AM, AACAP Work Group on Quality Issues: Practice parameter for the assessment of the family. J Am Acad Child Adolesc Psychiatry 2007; 46:922–937

Kollins SH: A qualitative review of issues arising in the use of psycho-stimulant medications in patients with ADHD and co-morbid substance use disorders. Curr Med Res Opin 2008; 24:1345–1357

Kratochvil CJ, Wilens TE, Upadhyaya H: Pharmacological management of a youth with ADHD, marijuana use, and mood symptoms. J Am Acad Child Adolesc Psychiatry 2006; 45:1138–1141

Libby AM, Riggs PD: Integrated substance use and mental health treatment for adolescents: aligning organizational and financial incentives. J Child Adolesc Psychopharmacol 2005; 15:826–834

March J, Silva S, Petrycki S, Curry J, Wells K, Fairbank J, Burns B, Domino M, McNulty S, Vitiello B, Severe J, Treatment for Adolescents With Depression Study (TADS) Team: Fluoxetine, cognitive-behavioral therapy, and their combination for adolescents with depression: Treatment for Adolescents With Depression Study (TADS) randomized controlled trial. JAMA 2004;292:807–820

March JS, Silva S, Petrycki S, Curry J, Wells K, Fairbank J, Burns B, Domino M, McNulty S, Vitiello B, Severe J: The Treatment for Adolescents With Depression Study (TADS): long-term effectiveness and safety outcomes. Arch Gen Psychiatry 2007; 64:1132–1143

Mensinger JL, Diamond GS, Kaminer Y, Wintersteen MB: Adolescent and therapist perception of barriers to outpatient substance abuse treatment. Am J Addict 2006; 15(suppl 1):16–25

Milberger S, Biederman J, Faraone SV, Murphy J, Tsuang MT: Attention deficit hyperactivity disorder and comorbid disorders: issues of overlapping symptoms. Am J Psychiatry 1995; 152:1793–1799

Singh MK, DelBello MP, Kowatch RA, Strakowski SM: Co-occurrence of bipolar and attention-deficit hyperactivity disorders in children. Bipolar Disord 2006; 8:710–720

Solhkhah R, Wilens TE, Daly J, Prince JB, Patten SL, Biederman J: Bupropion SR for the treatment of substance-abusing outpatient adolescents with attention-deficit/hyperactivity disorder and mood disorders. J Child Adolesc Psychopharmacol 2005; 15:777–786

Staton D, Volness LJ, Beatty WW: Diagnosis and classification of pediatric bipolar disorder. J Affect Disord 2008; 105:205–212

Upadhyaya HP: Managing attention-deficit/hyperactivity disorder in the presence of substance use disorder. J Clin Psychiatry. 2007; 68(suppl 11): 23–30

Weissman MM, Wolk S, Goldstein RB, Moreau D, Adams P, Greenwald S, Klier CM, Ryan ND, Dahl RE, Wickramaratne P: Depressed adolescents grown up. JAMA 1999; 281:1707–1713

Wilens TE: The nature of the relationship between attention-deficit/hyperactivity disorder and substance use. J Clin Psychiatry 2007; 68(suppl 11):4–8

Wilens TE, Faraone SV, Biederman J, Gunawardene S: Does stimulant therapy of attention-deficit/hyperactivity disorder beget later substance abuse? A meta-analytic review of the literature. Pediatrics 2003; 111:179–18

12

Substance Abuse

Get Me a Doctor Who Knows What He's Doing

VIGNETTE PART I

You are an attending psychiatrist on an adult inpatient unit. You receive a call from the hospital's intensive care unit asking you to admit a 22-year-old man 4 days after the patient overdosed on an unknown quantity of psychoactive medications plus an unclear amount of acetaminophen. The college roommate who found him unconscious estimated that the patient probably ingested the pills between 5 and 8 hours before admission; the patient was intubated for 24 hours at the beginning of the hospitalization but was soon able to breathe on his own. His serum acetaminophen level was 225 μg/ml, his aspartate aminotransferase (AST)/alanine aminotransferase (ALT) levels were 1,220/700 IU/L, and his urine toxicology screen was positive for opiates and cannabis. His blood alcohol level on admission to the emergency room was 0.28. His pupils were pin-point, suggesting opiate intoxication, and naloxone was administered. The medical team ordered that he be NPO and treated him with activated charcoal with gastric lavage and then began N-acetylcholine treatment over the next 72 hours and monitored him closely for the following 2 days. Normal saline, thiamine, and lorazepam, 1 mg i.v. every 2 hours, were administered during day 2 as the patient began to exhibit signs of acute alcohol withdrawal, including clouded consciousness, an inability to sustain attention, disorientation, and a core temperature of 39°C. He was treated for acute fulminant liver failure and responded quickly. According to the consultation-liaison (C/L) psychiatry resident who was called to see the patient on day 2, the patient continued to be delirious, irritable, agitated, and refused to speak, although he "kicked me out of the room." He noticed, however, a pack of cigarettes in the patient's belongings bag.

According to the patient's mother, whom the C/L psychiatry resident was able to reach by telephone on the opposite coast, the patient made two prior suicide attempts, both by overdose of medications, and had two subsequent inpatient psychiatric hospitalizations. She suggested checking his thighs for cut marks as he had engaged in self-mutilation off and on since he was at least 12 years old. He spent 2 weeks at an outpatient alcohol and substance abuse rehabilitation program in California when he was 16 after he was caught smoking marijuana at home. He attended 90 Alcoholics Anonymous meetings, attending daily for 3 months ("90 in 90") and then stopped going. He saw a psychotherapist sporadically from the age of 16 until he was 18 and was treated by a psychiatrist for major depression with fluoxetine 40 mg daily. He was accepted to a university in New York City.

When he was 6 years old he was sent by elementary school staff for a psychiatric evaluation because of inattentiveness and disruptive and impulsive behaviors. He was diagnosed with attention deficit hyperactivity disorder (ADHD). Methylphenidate was prescribed. However his mother said she and his father refused to give it to him because they were afraid it would cause him to become addicted to the drug. He continued to struggle in school, but managed to earn good marks because of his "natural intelligence." "He never had to study much," his mother told the resident. According to his mother, she is not sure if he is still using street drugs or if he still takes his fluoxetine because he does not call home more than two or three times a year, "and only when he needs money." She and her husband say their son does well in college and is due to graduate 1 year late after taking a year off to travel in Europe.

The lorazepam was slowly tapered beginning on hospital day 3 by 10%–15% per day. An antiemetic, non-opiate antidiarrhea formulation and fluids were administered or offered to help control the patient's withdrawal from opiates.

On hospital day 6 the medical team reports that the patient's vital signs have normalized, his acetaminophen level is 0, and his liver enzyme levels are moving toward normal limits, so you accept the transfer. The patient arrives several hours later, somewhat lethargic. He was given haloperidol 2 mg i.m. and lorazepam 1 mg i.m. by the treatment team after he learned he would be transferred to the psychiatry inpatient unit, had pulled out his intravenous lines, and left the hospital against medical advice. Six hours later, the patient is still lethargic, but his heart rate is 110 and blood pressure is 160/100 mm Hg. To control the patient's withdrawal symptoms, he was initially titrated to lorazepam 2mg every 4 hours. Prior to arrival on the inpatient psychiatric unit, the patient's lorazepam regimen had been tapered to 1.5mg every 4 hours, for a total of 9mg/day. The patient's vital signs normalize for approximately 4 hours, but he again becomes tachycardic and hypertensive.

DECISION POINT A

Given what you know about this patient's history of alcohol abuse and current symptoms, his refusal to speak with the resident, and not yet having spoken with him yourself, what would be the safest next step?

A1. _____ Until you are able to accurately assess the quantity and frequency of his alcohol abuse, you should not administer any additional pharmacotherapies. Wait until he is sober and able to provide a more detailed history to guide your decision making.

A2. _____ Until you are able to accurately assess the quantity and frequency of his alcohol abuse, you should not administer any additional pharmacotherapies. However, you should order aspiration precautions, ask nursing staff to provide visual cues to orient patient to time and place, and continue to monitor his vital signs every 2 hours for the first 12 hours and then every 8 hours. Apply a nicotine patch, 14 mg, and every 24 hours adjust according to symptomatology or to the patient's self-reported amount of smoking.

A3. _____ Continue the lorazepam taper by 10% every day. Tell the patient you noticed his cigarettes and offer him a nicotine patch to help withdrawal from cigarette smoking because smoking is not permitted in the hospital.

A4. _____ Order aspiration precautions because of the high dose of lorazepam, ask nursing staff to provide visual cues to orient the patient to time and place, and continue to monitor his vital signs every 2 hours for the first 12 hours and then every 8 hours. Start lorazepam 2 mg p.o. every 4 hours, holding the dose for sedation. Continue the taper by 10%–15% daily. Ask the patient if he would like a nicotine replacement therapy as he may be feeling agitated as a result of not smoking, which he cannot do in the hospital.

A5. _____ The patient is now out of the window for delirium tremens and his withdrawal symptoms are improv-

ing. Schedule him for outpatient follow-up within 3 days of discharge and give him chlordiazepoxide 50 mg tablets, 1 tablet every day for 3 days.

DECISION POINT B

Given what you know, how should you approach this patient?

B1. _____ Have the patient sign release of information forms to enable you to speak with his parents, psychiatrist, and therapist in California. Call each and obtain as much collateral information as you can.

B2. _____ Have the patient sign release of information forms to enable you to speak with his parents, psychiatrist and therapist in California. However, wait until the patient is more cooperative so you can explain what information you are seeking from these other sources.

B3. _____ Ask the patient to sit up and, if necessary, to splash water on his face so you can speak with him about the suicide attempt that led to this hospitalization.

B4. _____ If the patient refuses to speak with you, tell him he will not be going anywhere until he does. Explain that his suicide attempt was very serious, and you cannot allow him to leave the hospital in this condition.

B5. _____ Have the patient sign release of information forms to enable you to speak with his parents, psychiatrist, and therapist in California. Call each and obtain as much collateral information as you can. Ask the parents to fly to New York to participate in their son's treatment as he is abusing substances and the most effective strategy requires family work.

VIGNETTE PART II

You obtain consent from the patient to speak with his parents, his psychiatrist, and therapist in California. The patient is still refusing to speak with you about the suicide attempt. He asks repeatedly for "something to mellow me out" because "I'm really stressed and I'm going to explode." You explain that he is being carefully monitored for withdrawal symptoms, discomfort, and his lorazepam is being tapered. He becomes irate and screams, "Get out of my room! Get me a doctor who knows what he's doing. You are trying to torture me because that is what you get paid to do." Using a calm voice you explain again that the staff is carefully monitoring him, but you are unable to finish your sentence because he throws a shoe at you, which fortunately misses and hits the wall instead.

You contact the patient's mother who explains that she and the patient's father divorced 6 years ago after she caught him cheating with his legal secretary. She has one other child, a daughter, 20 years old, who attends a private college in northern California. The daughter briefly saw a therapist during the divorce. She was also diagnosed with ADHD when she was between 6 and 7 years of age; like her brother, she was never given the methylphenidate she was prescribed. She is not doing well in school, has a history of running away from home, using drugs, and underwent an elective abortion at the age of 15 after a rape.

The patient's mother suffers from depression and takes escitalopram. Her depression was diagnosed 1 year before the divorce. The patient's father allegedly has alcohol dependency that is untreated, but has not yet interfered with his ability to function as a malpractice attorney. She is not certain whether her parents had any psychiatric problems, but her father-in-law died of pancreatic cancer related to heavy drinking. She warns you not to call her ex-husband because he remarried, and has two young children and does not want to be involved.

The patient's former psychiatrist and therapist inform you that the patient's two previous suicide attempts, at ages 16 and 17, were probably related to his parents' divorce when he turned 16. They recall that the patient was diagnosed with ADHD by history that was not treated, but say he was lucky that he maintained good enough grades to move on to a university in New York. He had at least five episodes of major depression, beginning when he was 10 years old when he claimed that his father sexually molested him. The family was investigated by Child Protective Services, and no charges were made.

He again exhibited symptoms of depression at 12 and 15 years of age, the longest lasting 4 months, but his depression became disabling when he was 16, lasting more than 6 months and leading to his first suicide attempt. In between bouts of depression he says he felt "normal." During his depressions, however, he had anhedonia, was isolative, and ignored his friends. He typically lost 10% of his already lean body mass, had difficulty with sleep, and poor energy. After he was 16, he felt the divorce was his fault and continually ruminated with intrusive negative thoughts about himself. He never exhibited psychotic symptoms, homicidal ideation, or paranoid delusions. His mood was never elevated or euphoric, although he says it can change rapidly from "normal" to "really depressed." The mood switching can happen several times in a day and last a day or up to several months. There is no history of aggression toward people or animals, destruction of property, deceitfulness or theft, or serious violations of rules. He abused alcohol by binge drinking on weekends with friends beginning at the age 15. By the time his parents divorced, he was drinking by himself during the week as well.

His psychiatrist diagnosed him with "strong cluster B symptoms," but explains that he feels the patient's personality structure has taken on borderline personality disorder characteristics. By the time the patient was 12 it was noticed that he had begun cutting his thighs with a razor. The cuts were superficial, but there were numerous scars from his self-mutilation efforts and during visits typically six to eight fresh marks. None ever required sutures.

His friendships were of a fleeting nature. He would come to therapy or to see the psychiatrist extolling the virtues of his closest friends, but by the next month or two these friends had become enemies. Romantically, the patient seemed ambivalent about whether he preferred women or men and seemed to struggle with his own sexual identity. He often slept with strangers he met at bars, although he reported that he always used a condom. Even when he was in a better mood, he still complained of feeling empty, that his life was ruined, and he repeatedly blamed himself for his parents' divorce. He felt they may have set him up, to be the scapegoat for their decision to divorce by continually punishing him for alleged misconduct and poor grades, despite his "being the best son anyone could possibly want."

Therapy was started with fluoxetine 20 mg, which was increased to 60 mg over the next 4 months. He stopped taking the medication and seeing his therapist because he said he "felt fine" but again became depressed and made the second suicide attempt approximately 4 months later. He returned to the psychiatrist and therapist after a week-long hospitalization, and fluoxetine was restarted but was quickly titrated back to 60 mg. Again, once he felt better he quit coming to appointments and stopped the medication. He called the therapist one last time before leaving for New York.

His mother reported that he was excited to start at the university, felt good about his academic achievements, and seemed to have put the events surrounding his parents' divorce into better perspective. He acknowledged that their divorce had nothing to do with him or his sister; his father had cheated on his mother, and although he still harbored resentment toward his father, he told the therapist that he wanted to concentrate on his studies. She gave him referrals for a psychiatrist and therapist in New York City, but apparently he never followed up on them.

DECISION POINT C

Match the following drugs/substances with their approximate detection duration by urine toxicology screening:

1. Alcohol	A. 1–3 days
2. Amphetamines	B. ≤12 hours
3. Barbiturates	C. 48 hours
4. Cannabinoids (marijuana, hashish)	D. 2–3 days
5. Cocaine (coke, crack)	E. 8 days
6. LSD	F. 3–27 days
7. Opiates (heroin, morphine)	G. 1–7 days
8. Phencyclidine (PCP)	H. 1–5 days
9. Synthetic narcotics (China White, fentanyl)	I. 48 hours

VIGNETTE PART III

On hospital day 8 the patient has calmed down considerably and decides to speak with you. You ask him what precipitated the overdose. "I could not take it anymore," he tells you. "I have been lying to everyone to the point where I do not know which way is up. I am tired. I cannot handle all of the pressure anymore. I do not know what I'm going to do." His eyes become glassy and he grabs a few tissues. He tells you he is "pissed off" that his suicide attempt failed. When he sleeps he wakes up every hour or so and feels overwhelmed by his problems. He says he feels hopeless, helpless, and worthless. He cannot focus on anything, not even TV, and he has not been eating well. He apologizes for his behavior then blames the nursing staff for not helping him with PRN [as needed] medications. "You should fire half this staff," he tells you. "I've seen them do things to other patients that would get them arrested." You ask about his alcohol consumption. He tells you that he has been drinking on and off since the age of 12. "I can put away a fifth if I want." He began drinking by stealing sips of his father's drinks. He liked the way it felt and began stealing bottles from what he describes as "a huge bar." By the time he was 13 he was drinking 5 shots of vodka per night before bedtime. He would binge drink on the weekend and often blacked out, and "I ended up in some pretty odd places

doing some very odd things." He does not want to tell you about those incidents. He managed to maintain sobriety for 6 months when he started college, but this situation quickly deteriorated and he was again binge drinking. "My parents do not know this, but I was kicked out of school after my sophomore year." You ask what he has been doing for money and he replies that his parents send him large checks periodically "because I figure they owe me" and he also does "things" for money he prefers not to discuss.

You tell him you found evidence of opiates and marijuana in his urine toxicology screen. He admits to smoking marijuana infrequently, perhaps once per 1–2 months, only if someone "shoves a joint in my mouth." He does not use opiates, but overdosed on "a couple of handfuls of Vicodin" that his roommate had hidden because he sold the pills. "I do not get into that either," he says. "But I needed pills and they were around."

Regarding his general health, he reports that he is healthy, has had recent tests for sexually transmitted diseases including HIV infection, all of which were negative. In the past he contracted a chlamydial infection that was treated successfully with antibiotics. He says "the one thing I do right is practice safe sex." He says he smokes one pack of cigarettes per day and has smoked since he was 15 years old.

DECISION POINT D

Given what you know about this patient, what is your differential diagnosis? (+2) points for correct responses, including appropriate rule-out diagnoses, and (−2) points for incorrect responses.

Axis I:	
Axis II:	

DECISION POINT E

According to a meta-analysis of studies measuring the effectiveness of education and counseling to help patients make behavioral changes, no single intervention appeared more effective than others in changing behaviors, whether the purpose was to 1) add a behavior, 2) eliminate nonaddicting behavior, or 3) eliminate addicting behavior.

However, four strategies demonstrated the greatest change in promoting better health habits:

1. Rewarding the patient for positive behavior
2. Using multiple forms of information
3. Self-pacing and tailoring the intervention to the patient's needs
4. Providing feedback information about the change in health status measures.

Match the following variety of specific strategies for patient education and counseling with their corresponding definitions:

Strategy	Match the Definition
A. Shared-decision making	E1. _____ Addresses the patient's preconceived understanding of the effect of alcohol/substances on their health through a form of cognitive counseling delivered within a culturally sensitive fashion.
B. Social learning	E2. _____ Uses the power of peer pressures, mentorship, and social supports so patient does not feel alone in his or her addiction, is able to model more adaptive coping strategies, and can gain a sense of self-efficacy to fortify resolve to change his or her maladaptive behaviors. An example is Alcoholics Anonymous.
C. Health belief model	E3. _____ Uses interactive media (computer program, video, DVD) to show medical facts concerning the consequences of patient's behavior plus provides testimonies from patients who have made appropriate and healthy changes.
D. Cognitive behavioral therapy	E4. _____ Uses patient self-assessment questionnaires, logs of behaviors, triggers, emotions, goal setting, rewards, and functional analysis of drinking situations. Clinician use these data to help patients become educated about their addiction. A plan can then be developed to change behaviors.
E. Motivational interviewing	E5. _____ Uses the power of peer pressures, mentorship, and social supports so patient does not feel alone in his or her addiction, is able to model more adaptive coping strategies, and can gain a sense of self-efficacy to fortify resolve to change his or her maladaptive behaviors. An example is Alcoholics Anonymous.
F. Behavioral therapies	E6. _____ Focuses on positive reinforcement of desired behaviors, utilizing contracts and community reinforcements. Generally uses conjoint therapy, training in job finding, counseling focused on maintaining "sober" social contacts and environments and can be used to monitor adjunct pharmacotherapy such as disulfiram.
G. Marital and family therapies	E7. _____ Addresses alcohol abuse or dependence, with treatment goals that include stabilization of patient's social and interpersonal life, which may be considered as triggers for further abuse. Has not been well studied.
H. Psychodynamic and interpersonal therapies	E8. _____ Uses the dyad of husband and wife or the entire family system to better understand, cope with, and support the patient's treatment.

ANSWERS: SCORING, RELATIVE WEIGHTS, AND COMMENTS

High positive scores ($+3$ and above) indicate a decision that would be effective, would be required for diagnosis, and without which management would be negligent. Lower positive scores ($+2$) indicate a decision that is important but not immediately necessary. The lowest positive score ($+1$) indicates a decision that is potentially useful for diagnosis and treatment. A neutral score (0) indicates a decision that is neither helpful nor harmful under the given circumstances. High negative scores (-5 to -3) indicate a decision that is inappropriate and potentially harmful or possibly life-threatening. Lower negative scores (-2 and above) indicate a decision that is nonproductive and potentially harmful.

DECISION POINT A

The goal of treating this patient's acute alcohol and opiate intoxication as well as treating the overdose on acetaminophen were managed by the medical intensive care unit before the patient's transfer to the inpatient psychiatric unit. His withdrawal symptoms should decline sharply within the first 4–12 hours after his last drink and will peak in intensity by the 2nd day. He should begin to feel somewhat better by day 4 or 5. Symptoms include agitation, hyperactivity, anxiety, hand tremors, nausea or vomiting, insomnia, hallucinations or illusions with clear sensorium, tonic-clonic seizures, increased startle response, increased tendon reflexes, and orthostatic hypotension. Delirium tremens, a medical emergency, typically begins 48–96 hours, possibly up to 1 week after cessation of alcohol intake. This occurs in less than 5% of individuals and is heralded by the onset of delirium in most cases.

Like alcohol, opiates are short-acting; withdrawal from these substances is not likely to cause death. Patients typically experience withdrawal symptoms beginning from 6 to 24 hours after last dose, peaking at 48–72 hours, and lasting 7–10 days. This patient, owing to the context of overdose, was treated initially with naloxone, an opioid antagonist, to reverse the opioid effects. For treatment of mild to moderate withdrawal from opiates or maintenance therapy for withdrawal from opiates, patients typically can be treated with opioid agonists such as methadone, agonist/antagonists such as buprenorphine, or non-opioid agonists such as clonidine, an α_2-agonist antihypertensive drug that helps reduce insomnia, nausea, vomiting, diarrhea, muscle aches, and craving. Both buprenorphine and methadone are both metabolized by the liver, buprenorphine by one P450 enzyme and methadone by several P450 enzymes. Given the orthostatic hypotension caused by alcohol withdrawal, the emergency team chose to avoid clonidine. Studies have shown that buprenorphine is better tolerated and has greater acceptance for the treatment of mild to moderate opiate withdrawal by addicts. If the patient has ingested a high dose of opiates, buprenorphine can worsen the symptoms of withdrawal because of its antagonist properties. There are no well-designed studies at this time comparing buprenorphine with methadone, although methadone has also been shown to be very effective in acute withdrawal. Both buprenorphine and methadone are used for long-term stabilization and help with eventual cessation.

Nicotine withdrawal typically presents as a dysphoric or depressed mood, insomnia, irritability, frustration, or anger, anxiety, difficulty concentrating, restlessness, decreased heart rate, and increased appetite or weight gain. The symptoms and craving begin within 24 hours and decline gradually over a period of 10 days to several weeks. The patient is 6 days from his last cigarette and may be irritable and uncomfortable in part because of nicotine withdrawal. Offering him one of the nicotine preparations, such as Nicorette gum, the nicotine inhaler, or a nicotine patch would help alleviate these symptoms and help toward convincing the patient to quit smoking.

He is now 6 days free of alcohol and opiates and medically stabilized. His starting dose of lorazepam was 12 mg/day. He arrives on your unit with his lorazepam dose at 9 mg/day.

A1. _____ −5 This answer is incorrect because the patient requires some pharmacotherapy to manage his acute withdrawal from alcohol, opiates, and nicotine.

A2. _____ −2 This answer is incorrect regarding pharmacotherapy for the reasons explained in A1; however, adding environmental cues and aspiration precautions is helpful for a patient who has been delirious from hepatotoxicity, alcohol, and a drug overdose. The patient does not require such vigilant checking of his vital signs: every 8 hours is sufficient. Applying a nicotine patch is a good idea but should first be discussed with the patient and his permission should be obtained.

A3. _____ +2 Continuing the lorazepam taper by 10% per day and offering a nicotine patch are appropriate choices to help the patient's withdrawal from both alcohol and nicotine. However, the best answer should include aspiration precautions and monitoring vital signs for safety, and environmental cues to help the patient orient to time and place.

A4. _____ +5 This is the best answer.

A5. _____ −5 The patient should not be discharged for clear reasons of safety. He made a serious suicide attempt that has not yet been addressed, and he clearly is dependent upon alcohol. More history is required, and appropriate psychiatric follow-up must be arranged.

DECISION POINT B

B1. _____ +5 The only way to truly assess this patient, especially given his dependence upon alcohol and abuse of substances, is to gather collateral information.

B2. _____ −5 It is not necessary to wait to gather collateral information. You should not rely on the hope that the patient will become cooperative in a timely manner.

B3. _____ −5 This patient is recovering from his overdose and experience in the intensive care unit. You do need to learn about the suicide attempt, but an aggressive approach will probably ruin any chance of establishing a good rapport so he can comfortably speak about sensitive issues.

B4. _____ −5 Although it is true that the patient will probably remain an inpatient as long as he is unstable and uncooperative, and if you cannot establish a safe disposition, you should avoid the overly aggressive approach for the same reasons described in answer B3.

B5. _____ +2 Gathering collateral information will help you understand your patient better. Having the patient's parents join in the treatment process could lead to a better outcome. However, this depends entirely upon their current relationship and ability to fly from California to New York. Additionally, the two parents are not on speaking terms so this fact may further alienate one or both from the process.

DECISION POINT C

Score +2 points for each correct answer.

1. Alcohol	B. ≤12 days
2. Amphetamines	C/I. 48 hours
3. Barbiturates	G. 1–7 days
4. Cannabinoids (marijuana, hashish)	F. 3–27 days
5. Cocaine (coke, crack)	D. 2–3 days
6. LSD	A. 1–3 days
7. Opiates (heroin, morphine)	C/I. 48 hours
8. Phencyclidine (PCP)	E. 8 days
9. Synthetic narcotics (China White, fentanyl)	H. 1–5 days

DECISION POINT D

DIFFERENTIAL DIAGNOSIS

Axis I:	(+ 3) Major Depressive Disorder, recurrent, severe, without psychotic features (+ 2) Rule out Substance-Induced Mood Disorder (+ 2) Alcohol dependence (+ 2) Nicotine dependence (+ 2) Rule out marijuana abuse (+ 2) Rule out opiate abuse (+ 1) Rule out Bipolar Disorder
Axis II:	(+ 2) Deferred (+ 2) Strong cluster B traits (+ 2) Personality Disorder, NOS (+ 2) Borderline Personality Disorder

The patient arrives in your inpatient unit after a serious suicide attempt using an overdose in the context of heavy alcohol use. Subsequently, your initial evaluation may be complicated by whether this is a primary substance abuse or a dependence problem with subsequent mood symptoms or whether there is an underlying mood problem that is complicated by the dual diagnosis of a substance abuse or dependence diagnosis. Once you start to gather collateral information, and the patient begins to share more of his history, you learn that he has suffered at least five episodes of major depression beginning at 10 years of age, the longest lasting 6 months and ending with his first suicide attempt. He has been hospitalized twice previously for suicide attempts, has a history of self-mutilating behavior, and was diagnosed with ADHD as a child.

His current symptoms include disturbed sleep, feeling hopeless, helpless, and worthless, an inability to focus, and poor appetite. Because his mood symptoms preceded his abuse of alcohol and later substances by at least 2 years, it is likely that his mood symptoms underlie his substance and alcohol issues. Given that his major depressive episodes have lasted more than 2 weeks at a time, but less than 2 years, with symptom-free periods lasting greater than 2 months in between episodes, he can be diagnosed with Major Depressive Disorder, recurrent (+2 points). The severity of the symptoms, including suicide attempts, justifies the qualifier "severe," and he has not experienced any psychotic symptoms. Because the longest episode lasted 6 months, he does not qualify for Dysthymic Disorder (−2 points). However, given that this mood disorder did take place in the context of alcohol and substance abuse or dependence, one could write a rule-out for Substance-Induced Mood Disorder (+2 points).

Both he and his collateral informants have not endorsed any symptoms of mania or hypomania. However, when considering the early age at onset of depressive symptoms, the recurrence throughout adolescence, and the unclear family history (the father and paternal grandfather's alcohol dependence are strongly comorbid with mood disorders), it is not unreasonable to keep bipolar disorder as a ruleout. However, it would probably be lower on the differential (+1 point).

Given the earlier diagnosis of ADHD, this diagnosis could at least be carried over, listed as a ruleout, or listed in the patient's psychiatric history.

The differences between substance abuse and dependence as described by DSM-IV-TR are related primarily to the extent of disability caused by the use of this substance and the inability of an individual to cease using the substance:

This patient clearly has an alcohol dependency (+2 points) and a nicotine dependency (+2 points), but the evidence for making a diagnosis of cannabis abuse is not clear at this time other than the patient's admission he used it (but not frequently) and it showed up in his urine toxicology screen. Subsequently, a rule-out for cannabis abuse is warranted (+2 points). The patient used Vicodin (oxycodone-acetaminophen) tablets to overdose. He denies using opiates and claims he chose this drug because it was what he had available to him. Until we obtain a more detailed history of his opiate use we can write "rule out opiate abuse" (+2 points).

Table 1. CRITERIA FOR SUBSTANCE ABUSE

A. A maladaptive pattern of substance use leading to clinically significant impairment or distress, as manifested by one (or more) of the following, occurring within a 12-month period:

1. recurrent substance use resulting in a failure to fulfill major role obligations at work, school, or home (e.g., repeated absences or poor work performance related to substance use; substance-related absences, suspensions, or expulsions from school; neglect of children or household)

2. recurrent substance use in situations in which it is physically hazardous (e.g., driving an automobile or operating a machine when impaired by substance use)

3. recurrent substance-related legal problems (e.g., arrests for substance-related disorderly conduct)

4. continued substance use despite having persistent or recurrent social or interpersonal problems caused or exacerbated by the effects of the substance (e.g., arguments with spouse about consequences of intoxication, physical fights)

B. The symptoms have never met the criteria for Substance Dependence for this class of substance.

Table 2. CRITERIA FOR SUBSTANCE DEPENDENCE

A maladaptive pattern of substance use, leading to clinically significant impairment or distress, as manifested by three (or more) of the following, occurring at any time in the same 12-month period:

1. tolerance, as defined by either of the following:

    a. a need for markedly increased amounts of the substance to achieve intoxication or desired effect

    b. markedly diminished effect with continued use of the same amount of the substance

2. withdrawal, as manifested by either of the following:

    a. the characteristic withdrawal syndrome for the substance (refer to Criteria A and B of the criteria sets for withdrawal from the specific substances)

    b. the same (or a closely related) substance is taken to relieve or avoid withdrawal symptoms

3. the substance is often taken in larger amounts or over a longer period than was intended

4. there is a persistent desire or unsuccessful efforts to cut down or control substance use

5. a great deal of time is spent in activities necessary to obtain the substance (e.g., visiting multiple doctors or driving long distances), use the substance (e.g., chain-smoking), or recover from its effects

6. important social, occupational, or recreational activities are given up or reduced because of substance use

7. the substance use is continued despite knowledge of having a persistent or recurrent physical or psychological problem that is likely to have been caused or exacerbated by the substance (e.g., current cocaine use despite recognition of cocaine-induced depression, or continued drinking despite recognition that an ulcer was made worse by alcohol consumption)

Reprinted with permission from American Psychiatric Association: Diagnostic and Statistical Manual of Mental Disorders, 4th Edition. Text Revision (DSM-IV-TR). Washington, DC, American Psychiatric Association, 2000.

Table 3. DIAGNOSTIC CRITERIA FOR 301.83 BORDERLINE PERSONALITY DISORDER

A pervasive pattern of instability of interpersonal relationships, self-image, and affects, and marked impulsivity beginning by early adulthood and present in a variety of contexts, as indicated by five (or more) of the following:

1. frantic efforts to avoid real or imagined abandonment. **Note:** Do not include suicidal or self-mutilating behavior covered in Criterion 5.

2. a pattern of unstable and intense interpersonal relationships characterized by alternating between extremes of idealization and devaluation

3. identity disturbance: markedly and persistently unstable self-image or sense of self

4. impulsivity in at least two areas that are potentially self-damaging (e.g., spending, sex, substance abuse, reckless driving, binge eating). **Note:** Do not include suicidal or self-mutilating behavior covered in Criterion 5.

5. recurrent suicidal behavior, gestures, or threats, or self-mutilating behavior

6. affective instability due to a marked reactivity of mood (e.g., intense episodic dysphoria, irritability, or anxiety usually lasting a few hours and only rarely more than a few days)

7. chronic feelings of emptiness

8. inappropriate, intense anger or difficulty controlling anger (e.g., frequent displays of temper, constant anger, recurrent physical fights)

9. transient, stress-related paranoid ideation or severe dissociative symptoms

Reprinted with permission from American Psychiatric Association: Diagnostic and Statistical Manual of Mental Disorders, 4th Edition. Text Revision (DSM-IV-TR). Washington, DC, American Psychiatric Association, 2000.

This patient presents with a history that is very suggestive of Borderline Personality Disorder, and given his age, it is possible to diagnose this disorder. However, diagnosing personality disorders is very difficult if the clinician does not know the patient well, in the context of a severe mood disorder or episode, and in the context of substance abuse or dependence. If the underlying mood disorder is treated and the substance abuse or dependency issues are treated, and the patient still demonstrates a maladaptive personality structure, the diagnosis is much clearer. For this patient, given the long history taken from the patient and his mother, it is safe to label him as a rule-out Personality Disorder, not otherwise specified (+2 points), rule-out Borderline Personality Disorder (+2 points), or write "strong cluster B traits" (+2 points). The latter is not an official DSM-IV-TR diagnosis, but could help other clinicians who may treat this patient in the future. Writing "Deferred" is also appropriate if the clinician prefers to either wait to get to know the patient better and under sober and mood symptom-free circumstances (+2 points).

On axis II, the patient's admission that he has difficulty with interpersonal relationships, using black-and-white-type thinking, in which he is either "extolling the virtues" of his friends, or they are enemies. He describes mood lability, but no elevated or euphoric moods. He is easily irritable and demonstrates that while in the hospital. Finally, he has long demonstrated poor impulse control, using drugs, suicide attempts, self-injurious behaviors, ambivalence about his sexual identity, and relative sexual promiscuity. These personality traits have been enduring, and over the years have caused him to have interpersonal conflicts; in addition, the possibility that he was sexually molested as a young boy by his father led to an investigation by Child Protective Services. Subsequently, the patient meets criteria for Personality Disorder, not otherwise specified (+2 points).

Table 3 lists the DSM-IV-TR criteria for Borderline Personality Disorder.

DECISION POINT E

Score +2 points for each correct answer.

Strategy	Definition
C. Health belief model	E1. _____ Addresses the patient's preconceived understanding of the effect of the alcohol/substances on their health through a form of cognitive counseling delivered within a culturally sensitive fashion.
E. Motivational interviewing	E2. _____ Helps patient internalize the need to change his or her behaviors and move from reluctance and ambivalence to readiness and eagerness to change. Utilizes patient's intrinsic desire to change or enhances a patient's adherence to more intensive or extended treatment.
A. Shared-decision making	E3. _____ Uses interactive media (computer program, video, DVD) to show medical facts concerning the consequences of patient's behavior plus provides testimonies from patients who have made appropriate and healthy changes.
D. Cognitive behavioral therapy	E4 _____ Uses patient self-assessment questionnaires, logs of behaviors, triggers, emotions, goal setting, rewards, and functional analysis of drinking situations. Clinician use these data to help patients become educated a bout their addiction. A plan can then be developed to change behaviors.
B. Social learning	E5. _____ Uses the power of peer pressures, mentorship, and social supports so patient does not feel alone in his or her addiction, is able to model more adaptive coping strategies, and can gain a sense of self-efficacy to fortify resolve to change his or her maladaptive behaviors. An example is Alcoholics Anonymous.
F. Behavioral therapies	E6. _____ Focuses on positive reinforcement of desired behaviors, utilizing contracts and community reinforcements. Generally uses conjoint therapy, training in job finding, counseling focused on maintaining "sober" social contacts and environments and can be used to monitor adjunct pharmacotherapy such as disulfiram.
H. Psychodynamic and interpersonal therapies	E7. _____ Addresses alcohol abuse or dependence, with treatment goals that include stabilization of patient's social and interpersonal life, which may be considered as triggers for further abuse. Has not been well studied.
G. Marital and family therapies	E8. _____ Uses the dyad of husband and wife or the entire family system to better understand, cope with, and support the patient's treatment.

YOUR TOTAL

Decision Point	Your Score	Ideal Best Score
A		7
B		7
C		16
D		22
E		16
Total		68

KEY CLINICAL POINTS

1. Understanding withdrawal syndromes for abused substances will help the physician determine if a patient is in withdrawal, or is presenting with a primary psychiatric or medical illness.
2. To help determine a patient's apparent use or abuse, it is important to understand how long different psychoactive substances are detectable in a urine toxicology screen.
3. To best assess a patient with alcohol and/or substance abuse requires gathering collateral information.

REFERENCES

Azrin NH: Improvements in the community-reinforcement approach to alco-holism. Behav Res Ther 1976; 14:339–348

Bandura A: Social Foundation of Thoughts and Action: A Social Cognitive Theory. Englewood Cliffs, NJ, Prentice Hall, 1986

Chaney EF: Social skills training, in Handbook of Alcoholism Treatment Ap-proaches. Edited by Hester RK, Miller WR, New York, Pergamon Press, 1989, pp 206–221

DeBellis R, Smith BS, Choi S, Malloy M: Management of delirium tremens. J Intensive Care Med 2005; 20:164–173

DiMatteo MR. The Psychology of Health, Illness and Medical Care: An Individual Perspective. Pacific Grove, CA, Brooks/Cole, 1991

Dunn C, Deroo L Rivara FP: The use of brief interventions adapted from motivational interviewing across behavioral domains: a systematic review. Addiction 2001; 96: 1725–1742

Fiellin DA, Reid MC, O'Connor PG: Outpatient management of patients with alcohol problems. Ann Intern Med 2000; 133:815–827

Femino J, Lewis DC: Clinical Pharmacology and Therapeutics of the Alcohol Withdrawal Syndrome: Monograph 272. Rockville, Md, National Institute on Alcohol Abuse and Alcoholism, 1982

Gallant D: Alcohol, in The American Psychiatric Press Textbook of Substance Abuse Treatment, 2nd ed. Edited by Galanter M, Kleber H. Washington, DC, American Psychiatric Press, 1999, pp 151–164

Gordon GH, Duffy FD: Educating and enlisting patients. J Clin Outcomes Med 1998; 5:45

Higgins ST, Delaney DD, Budney AJ, Bickel WK, Hughes JR, Foerg F, Fenwick JW: A behavioral approach to achieving initial cocaine abstinence. Am J Psychiatry 1991; 148:1218–1224

Hodgson R: Treatment of alcohol problems. Addiction 1994; 89:1529–1534

Holbrook AM, Crowther R, Lotter A, Cheng C, King D: Meta-analysis of benzodiazepine use in the treatment of acute alcohol withdrawal. CMAJ 1999; 160:649–655

Holder HD, Longabaugh R, Miller WR, Rubonis AV: The cost effectiveness of treatment for alcoholism: a first approximation. J Stud Alcohol 1991; 52:517–540

Hunt GM, Azrin NH: A community-reinforcement approach to alcoholism. Behav Res Ther 1973; 11:91–104

Irvin JE, Bowers CA, Dunn ME, Wang MC: Efficacy of relapse prevention: a meta-analytic review. J Consult Clin Psychol 1999; 67–563–570

Mayo-Smith MF: Pharmacological management of alcohol withdrawal: a meta-analysis and evidence-based practice guideline. American Society of Addiction Medicine working Group on Pharmacological Management of Alcohol Withdrawal. JAMA 1997; 278:144–151

McClellan T, Dembo R: Screening and Assessment of Alcohol- and Other Drug-Abusing Adolescents: Treatment Improvement Protocol Series 3. Rockville, Md, U. S. Department of Health and Human Services, Center for Substance Abuse Treatment, 1993, p 116

Meichenbaum, D, Turk, DC: Facilitating Treatment Adherence: A Practitioner's Guidebook. New York, Plenum Press, 1987

Miller WR, Munoz RF: How to Control Your Drinking, revised ed. Albuquerque, University of New Mexico Press, 1982

Miller WR, Hester RK: Inpatient alcoholism treatment: who benefits? Am Psychol 1986; 41:794–805

Miller, WR, Rollnick, S: Motivational Interviewing: Preparing People to Change Addictive Behavior. New York, Guilford, 1991

Miller WR, Wilbourne PL: Mesa Grande: a methodological analysis of clinical trials of treatments for alcohol use disorders. Addiction 2002; 97:265–277

Monti PM, Abrams DB, Binkoff JA, Zwick WR, Liepman MR, Nirenberg TD, Rohsenow DJ: communication skills training, communication skills train-ing with family and cognitive behavioral mood management training for alcoholics. J Stud Alcohol 1990; 51:263–270

Price JL, Cordell B: Cultural diversity and patient teaching. J Contin Educ Nurs 1994; 25:163–166

Russell, ML: Behavioral Counseling in Medicine: Strategies for Modifying At-risk Behavior. New York, Oxford University Press, 1986

Sanchez-Craig M: Therapist's Manual for Secondary Prevention of Alcohol Problems: Procedures for Teaching Moderate Drinking and Abstinence. Toronto, Ontario, Canada, Addiction Research Foundation, 1984

Schwazzer R: Self efficacy, physical symptoms and rehabilitation of chronic disease, in Self-Efficacy: Thought Control in Action. Edited by Schwazzer R. Washington, DC, Hemisphere Publishing, 1992

Trevisan LA, Boutros N, Petrakis IL, Krystal JH: Complications of alcohol withdrawal: pathophysiological insights. Alcohol Health Res World 1998; 22:61–66

Can You Keep a Secret?

VIGNETTE PART I

You are a general adult psychiatrist in a private group practice in a small city, and your first appointment of the day is a new patient, Mrs. S. You received a summary from her most recent visit to the psychiatric emergency department at the local tertiary care hospital, with the patient's signed consent, that describes Mrs. S as "drug-seeking, most likely bipolar disorder II with psychotic features versus schizoaffective disorder."

Mrs. S arrives on time. On her intake form she wrote that her chief complaint at the moment is an inability to have sexual relations with her husband, whom she says wants a divorce because she is "frigid." She is somewhat conservatively dressed, her hair is pulled back into a bun, and she wears red horn-rimmed glasses with small clear crystals at the tips. She is obese and has apparent acne vulgaris on her cheeks, and she has good hygiene and is well groomed. You introduce yourself and offer your hand, but she seems not to have noticed and moves to sit in the chair opposite you; she immediately takes a tissue from the box on the coffee table. She is tearful and looking downward.

You take your seat on the other side of the coffee table and wait for her to gather her composure. A few minutes pass without her saying anything. Then she says, "I don't know why I'm here. It all seems so useless. I've been trying everything, and now John wants to leave me. It feels like I can't do anything right. He hates me." She begins to sob. She still has not looked up from the floor. You wait, but she does not offer any further information about what is so upsetting. Then she says, as if reluctantly, "I suppose you need a history, right?"

Mrs. S is a 35-year-old married woman with two adopted children, a 16-year-old son and a 15-year-old daughter, from her first relationship, which was not a marriage and which ended "amicably." She is still close to her previous partner, she says, and although he would

like to see his children, her current husband does not like him and will not allow him to come to the house. She was seen twice over 1 month in the local university's adult general psychiatry residents' clinic 2 years ago for a major depressive episode after a serious suicide attempt by overdose on acetaminophen. She recovered from the overdose without medical complications but remained depressed and anhedonic, with poor sleep, poor concentration, ruminating thoughts, and occasional impulsive behavior but no further suicide attempts. She had mild psychotic symptoms in the form of a non-command-type denigrating voice. She fired the treating resident at that time and did not return until recently, when she came to the hospital's psychiatric emergency room complaining of panic symptoms and suicidal ideation without intention or plan. She was not hospitalized, and she was referred to your clinic because she refuses to see another "inexperienced wannabe psychiatrist." She fired previous residents because she felt they were not responsive enough to her need for higher doses of benzodiazepines. Additionally, she admits to several visits over the past 6 months to three different medical emergency rooms with complaints of anxiety and panic.

She reports allergic reactions to lithium, fluoxetine, sulfa drugs, olanzapine, penicillin, and codeine. Her current medications include 60 mg of duloxetine daily, 20 mg of aripiprazole daily, and 0.5 mg of clonazepam twice a day. Previous medication trials included olanzapine, risperidone, lithium, fluoxetine, paroxetine, bupropion, buspirone, and alprazolam.

She completed all four modules of dialectical behavioral therapy in a group setting approximately 2 years ago and has had eight sessions with a master's-level therapist who used cognitive behavior therapy and supportive psychotherapy.

The patient has a history of opiate dependence after several surgeries, which included a cholecystectomy and several other operations that she adamantly refuses to discuss.

Her mother had major depression and anxiety and had made one suicide attempt; her older sister had major depression and had made two suicide attempts; her paternal grandfather had alcoholism and died 10 years ago of liver failure; and her father has alcoholism.

She currently lives with her husband of 2 years and the two children from her first relationship in a house just outside of town. She is a homemaker. Her husband works as a firefighter and is often not home for extended periods. They are financially stable.

Mrs. S makes herself comfortable in the chair opposite you and is no longer tearful. She says, "I don't know where to begin." She is looking at the framed medical credentials on your wall. "I've never had sex with my current husband." She again becomes tearful. You notice she grips the sleeves of her blouse with her fingertips. "He wants to. All the time, really. But I . . . can't. Or won't. No, I won't. I don't want to. I can't."

You wait.

"We never actually had sex in two years. I know that seems crazy. He understood for a while. We've been somewhat intimate, but I've never let him enter me. Now he wants a divorce, which I suppose is okay. I know I would want one if I were him. Look at me."

You ask if she was able to have sex in the past with her partner in her first relationship, and she replies that they did have sex, but it was "different." Then she looks directly at you and says, "Since you have a medical diploma from the university I'm going to trust you. I never told any of the other doctors any of this. Especially the residents, because they could not possibly understand. But I don't know what to do anymore. I don't want to lose my family, but I'm carrying a huge secret."

Before she will tell you, however, her tears resume, and she asks for a prescription for alprazolam, 1 mg t.i.d.

DECISION POINT A

Given the above information and presentation, what should you do? (Multiple answers are possible; points are taken away for incorrect answers.)

A1. _____ Continue to wait. She will continue to speak. You should not rush her, especially given her emotional lability. Demonstrate that you are concerned by placing a glass of water in front of her.

A2. _____ Begin the interview with an empathic statement such as, "I can see you are experiencing some emotional pain right now. I want you to know that everything that is said in this room will stay in this room, unless you are thinking of causing

harm to yourself or to someone else. In that instance I have a legal obligation to act on that information. Otherwise, it is OK to share anything you want with me."

A3. _____ Begin with an empathic statement: "I understand you were not entirely satisfied with your previous psychiatrist. Can you tell me why you chose to come here today?"

A4. _____ Since she is tearful, push the box of tissues closer to her and wait. Then begin by saying, "I received a note from your previous psychiatrist with a copy of your permission for him to share the information. I'd like to get to know you first, before I make any decisions about medications. You mentioned that you have a big secret you've been carrying around. You describe it in a way that makes me think it is a huge burden to you."

A5. _____ Tell her, "I received a note from your previous psychiatrist with a copy of your permission for him to share the information. I read some of the background, the medications you are currently on, and I must confess I am not likely to prescribe alprazolam in this context. However, I do want to help you. Let's start by your telling me in your own words what you expect from this visit."

DECISION POINT B

What are the four stages of the human sexual response cycle?

B1. Stage 1: _____

B2. Stage 2: _____

B3. Stage 3: _____

B4. Stage 4: _____

VIGNETTE PART II

Mrs. S becomes angry. "Are you going to be like all the other doctors? I came here for help. Are you going to tell me how to feel? Are you going to tell me everything is going to go away? Because it's NOT. You have NO idea." She continues to sob. "Xanax helps me. I know lots of doctors do not like to prescribe it to someone like me, but it HELPS."

You ask her how it helps.

"I get panic attacks. I can't control my anxiety. When I take a Xanax—which I don't abuse, I only use it when I need to—I feel better. Sometimes after I take it I end up having a panic attack anyway, so it's not the greatest medication. I can't sleep. All I do is worry about my husband, what he's going to think of me. . . ."

You wait.

"I'm a freak show, doctor. A real freak show." She gathers her purse and stands up. "I can't talk to you anymore about this."

You ask her why she feels the need to leave.

"If you aren't going to give me the medication, I'll have to find another doctor."

She starts to sob again and says, "I don't know if it's him or if it's me. Either way, I can't have sex. It's not that it's painful, I'm just afraid."

DECISION POINT C

Which agents affect the first three stages of human sexual response, positively or negatively? Fill in the appropriate boxes in the chart below using the list of agents provided. (Correct answers receive +2 points, incorrect answers receive −2 points.)

Stage of Response	Drug Classes That Have a Positive Effect	Drug Classes That Have a Negative Effect
Stage 1:_____		
Stage 2:_____		
Stage 3:_____		

- Selective serotonin reuptake inhibitors
- Anticholinergics
- Nitric oxide enhancers (e.g., sildenafil, which boosts cGMP action)
- Dopaminergic agents
- Dopamine receptor-blocking antipsychotics, some of which also increase prolactin
- Prostaglandins
- Beta-blockers (block noradrenergic function)
- Norepinephrine and dopamine reuptake inhibitors
- Dopamine-releasing stimulants (amphetamine and methylphenidate)

VIGNETTE PART III

Mrs. S states that she needs to tell you something that will help you understand her problem. She has not told you until now because she was not sure how you would handle the information, but she decided that you seem like an open-minded doctor and "this is too important," she says. "I am a postsurgical transsexual. I was able to have sex with my first 'husband' because at that time I still had a penis. He did not mind it when I started taking hormones and grew breasts, and he was even supportive when I had breast augmentation surgery. However, when I discovered that I would not be satisfied until I had sexual reassignment sur-

gery, he told me he could not maintain the same relationship with me." She smiles. "We're still friends, and he still sees the kids, but he is gay and wants to be with a man." She takes a deep breath. "I can live with that."

You ask if her new husband knows about her reassignment surgery. She says, "No. He actually thinks I'm a woman. I can't bring myself to tell him. My children know, but they're never around, so he never heard it from them. I don't know, maybe he did. But he never let on that he knows. Either way, he says he just isn't going to force me to have sex with him."

DECISION POINT D

Given the above information, what is your differential diagnosis for Mrs. S?

AXIS I:	
AXIS II:	

DECISION POINT E

Sexual dysfunction is divided into two primary disorders according to whether they describe a dysfunction of desire or of arousal. Use the following table to classify the listed criteria into one of the three columns.

Criteria	Sexual Desire Disorder	Sexual Arousal Disorder	Neither
E1. Inadequate lubrication-swelling response of sexual excitement			
E2. Recurrent or persistent involuntary spasm of the musculature of the outer third of the vagina that interferes with sexual intercourse			
E3. Recurrent delay in or absence of orgasm following normal sexual excitement phase			
E4. Persistently or recurrently deficient (or absent) sexual fantasies or desire for sexual activity			
E5. Persistent inability to attain, or maintain until completion of sexual activity, an adequate erection			
E6. No (or substantially diminished) subjective erotic feelings despite otherwise normal arousal and orgasm			
E7. Recurrent or persistent genital pain associated with sexual intercourse			
E8. Persistent or recurrent extreme aversion to, and avoidance of, all (or almost all) genital sexual contact with a sexual partner			

ANSWERS: SCORING, RELATIVE WEIGHTS, AND COMMENTS

High positive scores (+3 and above) indicate a decision that would be effective, would be required for diagnosis, and without which management would be negligent. Lower positive scores (+2) indicate a decision that is important but not immediately necessary. The lowest positive score (+1) indicates a decision that is potentially useful for diagnosis and treatment. A neutral score (0) indicates a decision that is neither clearly helpful nor harmful under the given circumstances. High negative scores (−5 to −3) indicate a decision that is inappropriate and potentially harmful or possibly lifethreatening. Lower negative scores (−2 and above) indicate a decision that is nonproductive and potentially harmful.

DECISION POINT A

A1. ____ +3 The patient is doing a fine job of relating her story. The best approach at this point is to listen carefully to what she says. This is obviously a complicated story. You should make notes about what areas seem to you worth further exploration in order to develop your differential diagnosis and consider what treatment options you would propose. Offering her a glass of water is a nice touch, but not necessary. Tissues should always be handy.

A2. ____ +4 A nice general empathic statement demonstrates that you are actively listening. Establishing formally for the patient that you will maintain her confidentiality is always important, and with this patient perhaps all the more so, given her feeling that her story may contain details that are especially distressing and involve her husband.

A3. ____ −2 This statement places you squarely in a competitive position with her previous psychiatrist. Asking why she chose to come today is an appropriate question, however.

A4. ____ +4 By offering the box of tissues and waiting, you are demonstrating both active listening and empathy through nonverbal communication, which at this point may be one of the more effective means of drawing the patient into a dialogue. After a period of waiting—which, as noted above in A1, is essential—you offer evidence that you took the time to get to know her case before she walked into the room. She will likely feel that you have made a reasonable effort to "do your homework" and be "ready" for her. You follow this with a more

specific empathic statement that will draw her attention to the specifics of the matter at hand. This may be too closed a statement, however. If you are concerned about time and wish to elicit what you believe to be highly sensitive information, a more effective possibility might be to use one of Shea's interviewing techniques, known as normalization, and say, for example, "Sometimes people who are harboring big secrets that affect their lives feel as though they are carrying a huge burden. This can impact their ability to function comfortably." You might also use another of Shea's techniques, such as gentle assumption, and suggest, "The secret you are carrying around seems to be impacting your relationship with your husband in an unhealthy way."

A5. ____ −3 While it is true that you have this information, sharing it in this way might cause her to become defensive. She has already expressed her disdain for psychiatrists who are unwilling to supply her with alprazolam. Your concern about a possible abuse of this medication is justified; however, if you wish to establish a good rapport with the patient, as well as a therapeutic alliance, you would be better served by listening to the story before judging her on the basis of other clinicians' experience.

DECISION POINT B

B1. ____ +2 Stage 1: Desire. Not dependent on physiological response, and is a reflection of the patient's motivations, drives, and personality; characterized by sexual fantasies and the desire to have sex.

B2. ____ +2 Stage 2: Excitement. Subjective sense of sexual pleasure and accompanying physiological changes; all physiological responses noted in Masters and Johnson's excitement and plateau phases are combined in this phase.

B3. ____ +2 Stage 3: Orgasm. Peaking of sexual pleasure, with release of sexual tension and rhythmic contraction of the perineal muscles and pelvic reproductive organs.

B4. ____ +2 Stage 4: Resolution. A sense of general relaxation, well-being, and muscle relaxation; men are refractory to orgasm for a period of time that increases with age, whereas women can have multiple orgasms without a refractory period.

DECISION POINT C

Correct answers receive +2 points, incorrect answers receive −2 points.

Stage of Response	Drug Classes That Have a Positive Effect	Drug Classes That Have a Negative Effect
Stage 1: Desire (libido)	Norepinephrine and dopamine reuptake inhibitors Dopamine-releasing stimulants (amphetamine and methylphenidate)	Dopamine receptor-blocking antipsychotics, some of which also increase prolactin
Stage 2: Excitement (arousal)	Nitric oxide enhancers Prostaglandins Dopaminergic agents	Selective serotonin reuptake inhibitors Anticholinergics
Stage 3: Orgasm		Selective serotonin reuptake inhibitors Beta-blockers

DECISION POINT D

Axis I:	Hypoactive sexual desire disorder (−2); sexual aversion disorder (+1); gender identity disorder (+2); rule out benzodiazepine abuse (+1); history of opiate dependence (+1)
Axis II:	Deferred (+2)

Hypoactive sexual desire disorder (−2). Since Mrs. S was able to have sex during her first relationship, the criteria of persistently or recurrently deficient (or absent) sexual fantasies and desire for sexual activity are not met. She did not describe a lack of desire for sexual activity but a fear that she will be "found out" by her husband, who does not know about how she has transitioned her sexual identity. It is reasonable to expect that if her husband accepted her sexual identity and was truly interested in having sexual relations with his wife, she would likely desire sex.

Sexual aversion disorder (+1). Mrs. S does avoid having sex with her husband out of fear that he will discover her transsexuality. Consequently, she persistently avoids all, or almost all, genital sexual contact with him. This disturbance clearly causes marked distress and interpersonal difficulty, as evidenced by her repeated attempts to find help from professionals and her husband's allegedly seeking a divorce. This sexual dysfunction might be considered better accounted for by her gender identity disorder if one considers only the interpersonal ramifications of keeping her transsexuality a secret from her husband. It is possible to specify subtypes of sexual aversion disorder to include acquired type, situational type, or due to psychological factors.

Gender identity disorder (+2). DSM-IV-TR criteria for this disorder include:

A. A strong and persistent cross-gender identification (not merely a desire for any perceived cultural advantages of being the other sex). It is manifested by symptoms such as a stated desire to be the other sex, frequent passing as the other sex, a desire to live or be treated as the other sex, or the conviction that he or she has the typical feelings and reactions of the other sex.

B. Persistent discomfort with his or her sex or sense of inappropriateness in the gender role of that sex. This is manifested by symptoms such as preoccupation with getting rid of primary and secondary sex characteristics (e.g., request for hormones, surgery, or other procedures to physically alter sexual characteristics to simulate the other sex) or belief that he or she was born the wrong sex.

C. The disturbance is not concurrent with a physical intersex condition.

D. The disturbance causes clinically significant distress or impairment in social, occupational, or other important areas of functioning.

Rule out benzodiazepine abuse (+1). From the interview so far, you have not been able to establish a more pervasive pattern to suggest substance dependence. The criteria for substance abuse, however, may apply on further evaluation. For this reason, the diagnosis is considered a "rule-out" until evidence is gathered. The criteria for *substance abuse* include:

A. A maladaptive pattern of substance use leading to clinically significant impairment or distress, as manifested by one (or more) of the following, occurring within a 12-month period:

1. Recurrent substance use resulting in a failure to fulfill major role obligations at work, school, or home (e.g., repeated absences or poor work performance related to substance use; substance-related absences, suspensions, or expulsions from school; neglect of children or household)

2. Recurrent substance use in situations in which it is physically hazardous (e.g., driving an automobile or operating a machine when impaired by substance use)

3. Recurrent substance-related legal problems (e.g., arrests for substance-related disorderly conduct)

4. Continued substance use despite having persistent or recurrent social or interpersonal problems caused or exacerbated by the effects of the substance (e.g., arguments with spouse about consequences of intoxication, physical fights)

B. The symptoms have never met the criteria for substance dependence for this class of substance.

Mrs. S has only described a need to obtain more alprazolam despite other physicians' refusal to prescribe adequate supplies. It is possible that she is using this medication to help with the anxiety caused by her marital discord. The primary maladaptive pattern she has suggested is "doctor shopping" for a clinician willing to prescribe a particular short-acting benzodiazepine known for its abuse potential. She has made this a central issue in her presentation despite the more substantial issues that she began to describe only later. For this reason, exploration of the above criteria is crucial to determine whether she has developed an abusive pattern of using this medication. You will be able to offer her safer methods for handling the stress she is experiencing both pharmacologically and psychotherapeutically once you establish an effective and positive therapeutic alliance. Given what you have learned of the experiences of her previous clinicians, you should be careful not to challenge her drug use early in the relationship, as this will drive her from your care.

History of opiate dependence (+1). From the history; there is no evidence of current use.

DECISION POINT E

Sexual dysfunction is divided into two primary disorders according to whether they describe a dysfunction of desire or of arousal. Use the following table to classify the listed criteria into one of the two categories, or neither.

Criteria	Sexual Desire Disorder	Sexual Arousal Disorder	Neither
E1. Inadequate lubrication-swelling response of sexual excitement		+2	
E2. Recurrent or persistent involuntary spasm of the musculature of the outer third of the vagina that interferes with sexual intercourse			+2
E3. Recurrent delay in or absence of orgasm following normal sexual excitement phase			+2
E4. Persistently or recurrently deficient (or absent) sexual fantasies or desire for sexual activity	+2		
E5. Persistent inability to attain, or maintain until completion of sexual activity, an adequate erection		+2	
E6. No (or substantially diminished) subjective erotic feelings despite otherwise normal arousal and orgasm	+2		
E7. Recurrent or persistent genital pain associated with sexual intercourse			+2
E8. Persistent or recurrent extreme aversion to, and avoidance of, all (or almost all) genital sexual contact with a sexual partner		+2	

Comments on the "Neither" answers

E2 describes a sexual pain disorder known as vaginismus. Dyspareunia, described in E7, is defined as recurrent or persistent genital pain associated with sexual intercourse in either a male or a female. E3 describes an orgasm disorder, of which there are male and female types. The primary difference between these types has to do with the wide variability in the type or intensity of stimulation that triggers orgasm in the female; otherwise they are essentially the same disorder.

YOUR TOTAL

Decision Point	Your Score	Ideal Best Score
A		11
B		8
C		20
D		7
E		16
Total		62

KEY CLINICAL POINTS

1. Two of the most effective techniques for establishing and maintaining an effective therapeutic alliance and subsequently help the patient to reveal sensitive information are empathy and validation.
2. It is important to understand the role of commonly prescribed medications and their effects, positive and negative, on human sexual response.
3. It is important to understand the difference between sexual desire and arousal disorders.

REFERENCES

American Psychiatric Association: Diagnostic and Statistical Manual of Mental Disorders, Fourth Edition, Text Revision. Washington, DC, American Psychiatric Association, 2000

American Psychiatric Association: Practice Guidelines for the Treatment of Psychiatric Disorders Compendium 2006. Washington, DC, American Psychiatric Association

Sadock BJ, Sadock VA: Synopsis of Psychiatry, 10th ed. Philadelphia, Lippincott Williams & Wilkins, 2007

Schatzberg AF, Nemeroff CB: Essentials of Clinical Psychopharmacology 2nd Edition. Arlington VA, American Psychiatric Publishing, 2006

Shea SC: The Practical Art of Suicide Assessment. New York, Wiley, 2002

Stahl SM: Essential Psychopharmacology. New York, Cambridge University Press, 2000

14

Gender, Race, and Culture

How to Exorcise in the Emergency Room

VIGNETTE PART I

You are the attending psychiatrist in the psychiatric emergency room at a tertiary care medical center on the East Coast of the United States. A woman is brought to the center by ambulance and wheeled in to the psychiatric emergency room strapped to a gurney. She is wrapped in a white linen shawl and is immobile. Although you are unable to see her face, you can see by her hands, which are tightly gripping the rails of the gurney, that she is dark skinned.

The paramedics report that they were dispatched to a private home in a nearby neighborhood after the patient's daughter called 911 because her mother was "shouting in a strange voice,"alternately with garbled speech and with strict demands that she be given specific items of clothing and jewelry. The daughter was reportedly anxious on the telephone and mentioned, "She's been acting strange

lately."The daughter has two children, a 4-year-old boy and a 2-year-old girl; her husband was not at home, so she told the paramedics she was going to take her children to a relative's house and then come to the emergency department.

The paramedics were unable to communicate with the patient because she spoke a foreign language and seemed unable to understand English. They had to use force to place her on the gurney, but she insisted with body language that her head be covered with the white shawl she had draped around her body. She apparently spat at them and seemed to curse, so they were happy to oblige. One of the paramedics tells you that she "seems possessed."She remained silent for the duration of the short trip to the hospital. She allowed them to take her vital signs and to perform a cursory physical examination; the findings were as follows:

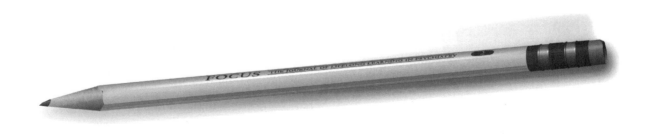

Blood pressure:	183/96 mm Hg
Pulse:	101 bpm
Temperature:	99.1°F
Head, eyes, ears, nose, throat:	Normocephalic; tattoo in the shape of a cross within a circle on the patient's forehead, apparently done many years ago given the faded quality of the thick dark inked lines. Unable to assess pupillary reflex or extraocular movements because the patient kept her eyes shut tightly. Unable to thoroughly assess mouth and throat except when the woman was screaming, at which time they noted that her oral mucosa seemed pink and moist and that her teeth had brown streaked discoloration. No thyromegaly, no lymphadenopathy.
Chest:	Clear to auscultation bilaterally without wheezes, crackles, or rales
Heart:	Regular rate and rhythm, S_1 and S_2 appreciated, no murmurs, gallops, or rubs
Abdomen:	Soft, nontender, no distension; bowel sounds appreciated; not hypo- or hyperactive
Extremities:	No clubbing, no wasting
Neurological:	Unable to assess as patient was not cooperative. From their struggles with the patient, they estimated that she had full strength in all four extremities and no obvious focal deficits

As you finish reading the notes on the physical examination, the patient begins to howl from behind her shawl. She struggles to free herself from the restraints and begins speaking loudly in what seems like pressured and hyperverbal speech, although in a language you do not recognize.

DECISION POINT A

Given the above presentation, what should you do? (Multiple answers are possible. Points are taken away for incorrect answers.)

A1. _____ Call for hospital security personnel to take the patient to a seclusion room, where she can be transferred from the ambulance gurney to a hospital gurney and kept in four-point restraints. Her behavior is disruptive, she is not redirectable, and she will likely agitate others in the waiting room. Since you do not speak her language and she is apparently psychotic, she will require medication with haloperidol

5 mg i.m. and lorazepam 2 mg i.m. to keep her calm until her daughter arrives to provide collateral information about her. Once the patient has calmed down, the restraints should be removed in a stepwise fashion, beginning with one wrist and the contralateral ankle. If the patient remains calm and the medications are sufficient, the remaining restraints should then be removed.

A2. _____ Call for hospital security personnel to take the patient to a seclusion room, where she can be transferred from the ambulance gurney to a hospital gurney and kept in four-point restraints. Her behavior is disruptive, she is not redirectable, and she will likely agitate others in the waiting room. Since you do not speak her language, you will wait for her daughter to arrive to provide collateral information about the patient.

A3. _____ Remove the patient's shawl from her face to examine her and attempt to communicate with her.

A4. _____ Do not remove the patient's shawl from her face to examine her and attempt to communicate with her.

A5. _____ Attempt to communicate with the patient through her shawl and explain that you understand she is experiencing a lot of frustration right now and you are taking her to a seclusion room until her daughter arrives. Ask if she understands you.

VIGNETTE PART II

You decide to place the patient in an isolation room but not in restraints. You do not give her any medications. Through your closed-circuit television monitoring system, you see that she is curled into a fetal position, wrapped in her white shawl, lying on the gurney, and quiet. After 20 minutes, the patient's daughter arrives. You bring her to an interview room, and she begins to sob. "I can't take this anymore," she says. "I brought her from Ethiopia last year because my father died and she did not have anyone to care for her. She is very traditional, but she has become very demanding lately. All I asked of her is to watch my children while my husband and I are at work during the day." She says that her children love their grandmother but find her strange because she has a tattoo on her forehead and they only understand some of what she says. "We've been trying to make the children bilingual by my only speaking to them in Amharic and their father only in English. But they are so young."

You ask her to describe her mother's behavior and how she thinks it has changed to the point where she required a trip to the psychiatric emergency room. The daughter explains that her mother seemed happy at first, but soon she became easily agitated, did not like to leave the house, hid upstairs when she and her husband had guests, and sometimes mumbled incomprehensibly to herself. About 3 weeks ago she demanded to be taken back to Ethiopia, but the daughter refused because there would not be anywhere for her to go there. "Besides, she was beginning to act more and more strangely, and I could not let her go back like that."

The daughter described her mother's behavior as increasingly agitated over the past 3 weeks, especially after she learned that she could not return to Ethiopia. She would often stay quiet for days, not uttering a word, and then would burst into screams, making demands in a strange voice, and acting as if she were possessed. The daughter clears her throat and looks around awkwardly. "I know you won't believe this, but there is a tradition in our culture called the *zar*," she says. "It is an evil spirit that supposedly takes possession of a person and makes them act somewhat like my mother has been acting. My experience with this is not extensive because I never actually saw someone "possessed,' but I heard from friends and older relatives that the possessed person does not necessarily become violent. My mother started throwing pots in the kitchen; she took some of my children's toys and hid them under her bed, and when she starts her screaming, she gets right in your face."

You ask if she believes her mother to be possessed by a *zar,* and if so, what is the remedy? The daughter replies that she does not believe in the *zar,* but "according to my limited knowledge, you have to have a coffee ceremony, find a *zar* exorcist, give the possessed person what they want, and if the spirit is satisfied, it leaves." She laughs uncomfortably and says, "I know it sounds crazy to you."

You reassure her that you are interested in the *zar,* that it is important in psychiatry to understand the person in order to understand the illness, and that you want to help her mother as best you can. The daughter then asks if she can see her mother.

Decision Point B

Given the above information, what should you do next? (Multiple answers are possible. Points are taken away for incorrect answers.)

B1. _____ Ask the daughter if she would be willing to translate for you, and bring her to her mother in the isolation room.

B2. _____ Ask the daughter if she would be willing to translate for you, but bring the mother to the interview room if she is cooperative.

B3. _____ Tell the daughter that hospital regulations prohibit her from coming back to the isolation room. Ask if she would be willing to translate for you, but ask her to sit in the waiting room until her mother is calm enough to be brought to an interview room.

B4. _____ Ask for the daughter's permission to give her mother medications, such as an anxiolytic or an antipsychotic, because of the behavior you have witnessed so far.

B5. _____ Ask the daughter for additional pertinent history, such as whether her mother had ever behaved in a similar way in the past, whether she has a previous diagnosis of mental illness, and about specific symptoms of depression, mania or hypomania, or psychosis.

Decision point C

List definitions for the following terms. (+5 points for correct answers.)

Term	Definition
C1. Ethnicity	
C2. Culture	
C3. Race	

VIGNETTE PART III

The patient refuses to move. You call the hospital's translation service and ask for an Amharic translator. (Alternatively, you ask the daughter if she knows of any members of the Ethiopian community who are not related to her family who may be willing to translate, and then ask for assistance.) You bring the daughter to the isolation room. She approaches her mother, strokes her head, and speaks to her in Amharic. The mother does not respond. The daughter continues to speak to her until her mother abruptly speaks in a strange, deep-tenor voice. You ask the daughter to tell you precisely what her mother is saying, word for word. "She's just saying, 'I need coffee. I need coffee. I will not release her until you bring me coffee and a new dress.' See?" She shrugs. "She's lost it. She's pretending to be possessed. I'm supposed to go and buy her a dress on a Friday night? Is she crazy?"

The patient begins to rattle the rails of the gurney and starts screaming. The shawl has come off her face, and you see she has her eyes closed. Then she opens them and looks around, but continues screaming. The daughter backs up and leaves the room.

DECISION POINT D

Given everything you have learned to this point, what is your differential diagnosis?

Axis I:	
Axis II:	

DECISION POINT E

The Outline for Cultural Formulation contained in DSM-IV-TR is "meant to supplement the multiaxial diagnostic assessment and to address difficulties that may be encountered in applying DSM-IV-TR criteria in a multicultural environment." What are the five parts of the cultural formulation?

E1. _____
E2. _____
E3. _____
E4. _____
E5. _____

VIGNETTE PART IV

The patient is given haloperidol 2 mg i.m. and lorazepam 2 mg i.m. After an hour she is calm but alert. Her daughter continues to translate. You learn that the patient is oriented to person, place, and time, but she still lapses into a strange-sounding voice, which the daughter refers to as her mother's *zar*. When speaking in this voice, the patient is demanding a coffee ceremony, a dress, and to be taken back to Ethiopia. Your assessment is that the patient is acutely psychotic, and you admit her to the inpatient psychiatry unit for safety and further evaluation. She is started on risperidone, which is titrated to 3 mg daily. She is also started on sertraline, which is titrated to 150 mg daily for mood symptoms. After 1 week, the patient is no longer agitated and she sleeps well, but she still lapses into her "possessed voice" several times each day.

You are now the treating psychiatrist on the inpatient floor. You do not find an available Amharic speaking translator, so you depend on the daughter for communication with the patient and for collateral information. You use the Internet to learn about the *zar*, which is described as a culturally based syndrome common to certain countries in Africa, including Ethiopia. The *zar* functions in a wide range of crisis-oriented contexts, including infertility, role clashes, marriage difficulties, and intense social and cultural change. *Zar* illness and therapy, therefore, can represent a method of coping with a disruptive condition, whether it is physiological, psychological, or social. When an individual is afflicted with a *zar*, he or she attends a *zar* ceremony with others who have experienced similar illness. A trance is induced, and the *zar* spirit then enters the person's body and reveals its identity and wishes through movement and speech. The spirit is not exorcised; rather, the individual forms a relationship with it to prevent future episodes of illness. This typically requires that the individual accept "to undertake certain activities, which may include performing certain rituals, attending regular *zar* ceremonies, wearing special clothing or jewelry, ingesting specific foods or other substances such as tobacco, or altering his or her marital status to appease the spirit"(Edelstein 2002).

After 10 days, the daughter tells you that she is willing to take her mother home but believes she needs outpatient psychiatric care.

DECISION POINT F

Given what you know about the patient's progress on the inpatient unit and what you learned by developing a cultural formulation of the case, what are the most appropriate steps for you to take to help this patient? (Multiple answers are possible. Points are taken away for incorrect answers.)

F1. _____ The patient is likely depressed and anxious. She may be using the *zar* to express her mental distress. Continue her antidepressant medication, but wean her from the antipsychotic before discharge, as she probably does not need it. Hold the patient in the inpatient unit until you are able to find an Amharic-speaking therapist in the community for outpatient psychotherapy.

F2. _____ Discharge the patient to her daughter's care, since she has agreed to take her mother home. Continue the risperidone and sertraline at the dosages prescribed in the hospital, since she is tolerating them well.

F3. _____ The patient is suffering from a culturally based syndrome, and medications are useless. Discontinue the risperidone and sertraline. Discharge the patient to her daughter's care, since she has agreed to take her mother home.

F4. _____ Arrange to have a person from the Ethiopian community visit the hospital and perform a *zar* ceremony to help the patient through her crisis according to the tradition. Then discharge her to her daughter's care if she improves.

F5. _____ Arrange a *zar* ceremony yourself on the basis of what you learn about the tradition, with help from the daughter's family. If the ceremony works and the patient improves, discharge her to her daughter's care.

ANSWERS: SCORING, RELATIVE WEIGHTS, AND COMMENTS

High positive scores (+3 and above) indicate a decision that would be effective, would be required for diagnosis, and without which management would be negligent. Lower positive scores (+2) indicate a decision that is important but not immediately necessary. The lowest positive score (+1) indicates a decision that is potentially useful for diagnosis and treatment. A neutral score (0) indicates a decision that is neither clearly helpful nor harmful under the given circumstances. High negative scores (−5) indicate a decision that is inappropriate and potentially harmful or possibly life-threatening. Lower negative scores (−2 and above) indicate a decision that is nonproductive and potentially harmful.

DECISION POINT A

A1. _____ +2 While this exercise is designed to explore how a clinician should approach a patient whose cultural expression of illness may be in question or whose language the clinician does not understand, the first rule in the emergency department regarding a patient who is agitated and not redirectable is to stabilize the patient and the situation. According to the narrative, the patient is so agitated that there should be concern about placing her with other patients in the waiting room. It is important to control the acuity level in the waiting room, so removing the patient to a seclusion room in this instance makes sense. Giving the patient haloperidol 5 mg i.m. and lorazepam 2 mg i.m. represents the standard of care in treating a patient who is agitated and not redirectable. However, since you do not understand her, a diagnosis of psychosis may or may not be appropriate. Behavioral dyscontrol seems more apparent. In this case, the restraints were necessary to transfer the patient to the hospital and then to the seclusion room.

A2. _____ −3 Removing the patient to a quiet area and awaiting her daughter's arrival are appropriate steps, but use of physical restraints alone is not. Standard of care is to avoid the use of physical restraints when possible and to use chemical restraints first. Medications should be the first-line option for controlling this patient's agitation, even if she is already in physical restraints for the transfer to the seclusion room.

A3. _____ +5 You must perform at least a cursory physical examination of this patient to rule out any obvious signs of trauma or potentially reversible causes of her dyscontrol. Now that you are the physician responsible for her care, you cannot rely on the report from the paramedics' examination. You may be concerned about offending the patient by removing her shawl, looking into her eyes, and touching her in any way or offending her in some other unintended way. For this reason (especially if you are a male physician), it is a good idea to have a female nurse or other clinician with you while you perform the examination.

A4. _____ −5 As stated above, you must perform at least a cursory physical examination of the patient. While it is possible that you will offend her by removing the shawl, you are a medical professional with a duty to care for this patient. The paramedics told you that the patient's daughter expects to arrive at the hospital soon, but you have no way of knowing when she will arrive.

Since the patient is acting in a way that suggests a need for emergent treatment, you must evaluate her immediately.

A5. _____ +3 Attempting to communicate, explaining your actions despite your uncertainty about whether the patient understands you or not, and taking her to a seclusion room because of her dyscontrol are all appropriate actions.

DECISION POINT B

B1. _____ +5 You must make every attempt to communicate with your patient. The daughter represents your best opportunity to learn both from the patient and about the patient from a collateral source. If your hospital lacks an appropriate translator or is unable to find one who can help at this instant, you must use the resources available—in this case, the daughter. Keep in mind that she will likely interpret more than translate, since she is the patient's daughter, lives with the patient, and was the source of the 911 call that brought the patient to the emergency department. You should interview the daughter separately, just as you would with any family members who come in with a patient, especially since the patient is unable or unwilling to respond.

B2. _____ +3 It would be more comfortable for the patient if she could move from the isolation room to an interview room. However, this would require that you be able to communicate with the patient in some fashion to ascertain whether she understands you. Given the patient's acute presentation and the circumstances in the emergency room, this might not yet be possible.

B3. _____ −5 If the daughter is your sole means of communicating with this patient, she should be brought to the isolation room if necessary. You should find the most effective means to evaluate the patient emergently.

B4. _____ +3 Since your patient is unable to communicate directly with you, you require the daughter's help to evaluate the patient. If the daughter is able to translate and the patient is responding appropriately to your questions and it is apparent that she understands you, you can ask her permission to provide treatment if you deem it necessary. If the patient remains unable to communicate and you conclude that it is necessary to medicate her, you can give emergent medications without consent.

B5. _____ +5 As stated in B1, you need collateral information about the patient. Since the daughter is there, you should see what you can learn from her about your patient, keeping in mind that she is a biased source. You can research cultural differences or expressions of illness unique to your patient later, once the patient is stabilized.

DECISION POINT C

Term	Definition[a]
C1. Ethnicity	(+5) Identification with, and feeling part of, an ethnic group, and exclusion from certain other groups because of this affiliation.
	Ethnic group: Group distinguished by cultural similarities (shared among members of that group) and differences between that group and others; ethnic group members share beliefs, values, habits, customs, and norms and a common language, religion, history, geography, kinship, and/or race.
C2. Culture	(+5) Distinctly human; transmitted through learning; traditions and customs that govern behavior and beliefs.
C3. Race	(+5) Can be broken down into biological and social race. This question is about social race: a group assumed to have a biological basis but actually perceived and defined in a social context, by a particular culture rather than by scientific criteria.

[a]From Conrad, 2006

DECISION POINT D

Axis I:	Psychotic disorder not otherwise specified (+2); rule out malingering (+2); rule out dissociative trance disorder (+2)
Axis II:	Deferred (+2)

The patient is displaying psychotic symptoms in the form of disorganized speech, behavior, and possible delusions or hallucinations. While it may be possible to explain her behavior and speech from a cultural perspective, at the moment it is not possible to independently validate the daughter's translation or accept her interpretations. Moreover, the patient may be psychotic and expressing her symptoms in a way that is culturally familiar to her. For now, without further evidence or information to make a specific diagnosis, the more nonspecific diagnosis of psychotic disorder not otherwise specified is appropriate.

Once the patient is stabilized, you should find an objective translator and conduct research on the *zar*. If you consider the patient's alleged possession by a *zar* a cultural expression of illness, to label her symptoms as malingering would be the same as denouncing the *zar* as intentional. If the patient is using the *zar* intentionally, then malingering is appropriate. Otherwise, the *zar* can be considered a dissociative disorder, specifically a dissociative trance disorder, which is defined as single or episodic disturbances in the state of consciousness, identity, or memory that are indigenous to particular locations and cultures. According to DSM-IV-TR, dissociative trance involves narrowing of awareness of immediate surroundings or stereotyped behaviors or movements that are experienced as being beyond one's control. Possession trance involves replacement of the customary sense of personal identity by a new identity, attributed to the influence of a spirit, power, deity, or other person and associated with stereotyped "involuntary" movements or amnesia.

Because you are a Western doctor in a Western hospital, it is appropriate to use psychotic disorder not otherwise specified as the primary diagnosis and dissociative trance disorder as the rule-out.

DECISION POINT E

E1. ____ +2 **Cultural identity of the individual.** This patient is an Amharic-speaking Ethiopian. She is unable to speak English. She recently immigrated to the United States. The tattoo on her forehead suggests that she is or was significantly involved with her culture of origin. Additional information about the patient's religion, her culture of origin, her level of participation in her religion or culture, and the context of this level of participation would help in the evaluation.

E2. ____ +2 **Cultural explanations of the individual's illness.** This patient presents as possibly being possessed by a *zar,* which is described in the DSM-IV-TR Glossary of Culture-Bound Syndromes (in the same appendix as the Outline for Cultural Formulation). It is important to obtain information about the patient's pref-

erences for and past experiences with professional and popular sources of care.

E3. ____ +2 **Cultural factors related to psychosocial environment and levels of functioning.** This patient is unable to communicate outside her home, has no significant social supports other than her daughter and immediate family, and is living in a country with which she is unfamiliar, far from the comfort of her culture of origin. It is important to understand how the patient and her family experience death and bereavement, given that the patient lost her husband within the past year.

E4. ____ +2 **Cultural elements of the relationship between the individual and the clinician.** You do not speak Amharic, so direct oral or written communication is impossible. She is not responding to you, possibly because she is frightened, unfamiliar with the environment of your emergency room, and/or shaken by having been brought here forcibly—all of which are added on top of the issues that elicited the 911 call in the first place. She does respond to her daughter, although it seems apparent that there are some interpersonal difficulties between them, so accurate evaluation without the help of an impartial translator is problematic. Her behavior is possibly within the realm of a cultural syndrome. There may be social norms for interaction between unmarried members of the opposite sex about which you are unaware. Until you learn enough about how your patient would expect you to behave in a similar context based in her culture of origin, you will not know if you are unintentionally creating barriers between you and the patient.

E5. ____ +2 **Overall cultural assessment for diagnosis and care.** Whether or not this patient's symptoms are related directly to her possession by a *zar,* she meets the diagnostic criteria for being psychotic, her behavior is unpredictable, erratic, and violent, and you cannot determine with any certainty whether she is a risk to herself or to others. If she is not able to calm down even with the help of her daughter, she should be given an antipsychotic and an anxiolytic, either orally or, if she does not cooperate, by injection. Given the severity of her symptoms, you would admit her to a psychiatric inpatient facility. You will need an Amharic translator if available.

DECISION POINT F

F1. ____ +3 There are many psychosocial stressors that may have caused this patient to become depressed and anxious. She may be expressing her mental distress according to an acceptable culturally based syndrome and not actually be psychotic. While she is in the safe environment of the inpatient unit, an attempt to wean her from the antipsychotic may be appropriate, especially given the physiological risk and the cost of these medications. However, waiting for an Amharic-speaking therapist before discharging the patient is not practical. This patient, if your assessment is correct, would benefit from individual psychotherapy to cope with her many psychosocial stressors. However, finding an Amharic-speaking therapist may be difficult or impossible. Arranging follow-up at an outpatient psychiatric clinic with the daughter present may be the best you can do. It may not be possible to accommodate the most culturally appropriate treatment.

F2. _____ +3 As stated above, you may not be able to accommodate the most culturally appropriate treatment for the *zar*, so you continue to treat the patient according to your working differential, which includes psychosis. You may wish therefore to keep this patient on risperidone for now and consider weaning her from it during outpatient treatment after she is discharged. If the patient is not truly psychotic, you will want to minimize the use of the antipsychotic because of the physiological risk and the cost.

F3. _____ −3 Although this may be true, you are responsible for the patient, and until it is possible to better evaluate her, simply stopping the medications and sending her home may cause a relapse of the more violent and unpredictable symptoms and put the patient and her family in danger.

F4. _____ +3 This is ideal, although given the information you have, it seems unlikely that it will occur.

F5. _____ −3 This is probably not feasible or advisable.

YOUR TOTAL

Decision Point	Your Score	Ideal Best Score
A		10
B		16
C		15
D		8
E		10
F		9
Total		62

KEY CLINICAL POINTS

1. In the conceptualization of a patient, Ethnicity, Culture, and Race have specific and different meanings; the physician's conceptualization of a patient may affect approach to treatment.
2. The five part cultural formulation included in the DSM-IV-TR supplements the multiaxial diagnostic assessment and addresses difficulties that may be encountered in applying DSM criteria in a multicultural environment.
3. Although a patient's presentation may be culturally-based, it is appropriate to use western-based approaches to assess safety and treat accordingly.

REFERENCES

American Psychiatric Association: Diagnostic and Statistical Manual of Mental Disorders, Fourth Edition, Text Revision. Washington, DC, American Psychiatric Association, 2000

American Psychiatric Association: Practice Guidelines for the Treatment of Psychiatric Disorders Compendium 2006. Arlington VA, American Psychiatric Association, 2006

Conrad PK: Cultural Anthropology, 11th ed. New York, McGraw-Hill, 2006

Edelstein M: Lost tribes and coffee ceremonies: Zar spirit possession and the ethno-religious identity of Ethiopian Jews in Israel. J Refug Stud 2002; 15:153–170

Sadock BJ, Sadock VA: Synopsis of Psychiatry, 10th ed. Philadelphia, Lippincott Williams & Wilkins, 2007

SEROTONIN SYNDROME

Author Note: a good point that merits some discussion.

In the table of answers for Decision Point E, we did not include autonomic dysfunction as a necessary sign or symptom of serotonin syndrome. However, serotonin syndrome can present with autonomic dysfunction and is considered a medical emergency. The more serious effects of serotonin syndrome can be life threatening.

Although serotonin syndrome is likely underreported because of the teeming differential diagnoses of delirium tremens, heatstroke, stiff man syndrome, sepsis, poisoning by overdose of sympathomimetic or anticholinergic agents, and (as noted in the exercise) the common symptoms of neuroleptic malignant syndrome.

Serotonin syndrome is less likely today than in the past to have a bad outcome, at least according to the sparse literature, largely because of the general drop in the use of monoamine oxidase inhibitors, which, when combined with any medication that would rapidly increase serotonin levels, would cause hyperreflexia, myoclonus, muscular rigidity, hyperthermia, and autonomic instability. Nevertheless, the potential development of serotonin syndrome certainly should be watched closely, especially when augmentation strategies are used in treatment with antidepressants or when serotonergic sleep aids are added.

In a case of severe serotonin syndrome, initial treatment with benzodiazepines and cyproheptadine (an an-tihistamine with serotonin antagonist properties) is appropriate. One must also be ready for endotracheal intubation to protect the airway if muscular rigidity, hyperthermia, or neuromuscular paralysis do not respond to initial treatment.

15

Psychotherapy

Why Must You Be Such an Angry Young Man?

VIGNETTE

You are a psychiatrist in private practice. A 20-year-old male patient was discharged from the psychiatric inpatient unit at the local university hospital 5 days ago and was referred to you for follow-up. He had been hospitalized for 7 days after he was involved in a motor vehicle accident. In the field sobriety test, he registered 0.08 on the Breathalyzer, and he was cited for driving under the influence of alcohol. He had a court date set for his DUI in 2 weeks, and his attorney said he would likely be sentenced to 1 year of probation. When he was brought to the emergency department for treatment of a broken wrist and numerous lacerations, he announced that he was suicidal. After he received treatment for his injuries, he was transferred to the psychiatric emergency room, where he was evaluated and admitted for treatment of major depression with suicidal ideation.

According to his self-reported history, he had trials of fluoxetine, paroxetine, lithium, divalproex, haloperidol, olanzapine, risperidone, clonazepam, lorazepam, and possibly other medications that he is unable to recall. He was not very clear on how long he was on each medication, nor precisely why he stopped each one. He just said that the drug didn't work, or said that it made him gain 30 pounds, or said "I have no idea."

During his stay on the inpatient unit, he was combative with staff, and he had to be placed in the isolation room three times for 4-hour periods because of violent threats and an attempt to harm himself with a plastic utensil he had stolen from the dining room. On one occasion he banged his head repeatedly against the wall in the bathroom, creating a laceration that required three stitches. He was given a lorazepam taper for the first 5 days to protect against withdrawal symptoms, and he was given haloperidol injections during his outbursts. To treat his depression, he was given fluoxetine,

titrated to 40 mg by the end of his stay. He was also started on 100 mg of trazodone at bedtime for insomnia.

By day 6 of his hospital stay, he had calmed down considerably, participated in groups, and expressed a great deal of remorse about his behavior. By day 7, he was considered safe from suicidal thoughts and well enough to be discharged.

He arrives early for his appointment with you. When he enters your office, you observe that he is dressed in a suit and his hair is meticulously groomed. He has a cast on his right forearm and wrist. He is very polite and appears calm.

He takes his seat and you begin the interview. He tells you that his father passed away 2 months earlier after a 5-month battle with a neoplastic blood disorder that was not diagnosed appropriately in the hospital. Although he is unable to provide any details, he says that mistakes were made regarding his father's treatment in the hospital that may have contributed to his death. He tells you that the hospital's vice president visited the family to offer his apologies.

He was very close with his father, and his death affected him deeply. He had moved 7 months ago from his family's previous hometown to be with his father in the hospital. Before that he had been unemployed, living with his mother. He did not continue school after graduating from high school. At first he stayed with his brother, who attends the local university, and then moved in with his mother after she took an apartment close to the hospital. While his father was in the hospital, the patient began drinking vodka from a flask he carried. He said he would step into the bathroom frequently and take nips from the flask and go out to the parking lot to refill it; soon he was drinking a fifth of vodka per day. Before that, he had been sober for 1 year from alcohol dependence, which he started abusing at age 16, although he continued to smoke marijuana daily, which he had also started at 16.

He has been in several inpatient and outpatient substance rehabilitation programs. He had attended AA meetings in the past and found them very helpful, but his father's illness caused him to relapse. He says that he has smoked marijuana consistently during the past 4 years, increasing the amount he smoked from one joint at night before bedtime to about a quarter ounce per week. He spent a great deal of time finding ways to obtain marijuana, and although he wanted to stop using the drug, he was unable to. "I was losing my memory," he said, "and I lost the desire to do anything with my life." He had frequent fights with his mother about his marijuana use: "She kept sticking me in rehab." Since age 16 he has also abused crack cocaine, powder cocaine, LSD, psilocybin mushrooms, and γ-hydroxybutyrate (GHB). "Pretty much anything anyone had, I would do," he says.

He did very poorly in high school, although he did manage to graduate, and he enrolled in a few classes at his local community college before his father was hospitalized. He did not complete the courses, however; he could not get himself to go to class for fear of what others thought of him, and then he moved to be with his father. You ask him what he considers to be his biggest issue, and he replies, immediately, "Anger." He explains that since the age of 14 he has increasingly been involved in physical fights, many involving injuries: he has sustained broken bones, he has a torn tendon and nerve damage in one hand that limits his ability to use two of his fingers, and his left shoulder easily dislocates. He has an appointment with an orthopedic surgeon to correct the shoulder problem in 2 months' time.

You ask about legal issues, and he tells you he was taken to juvenile court at age 14 for "setting the woods on fire. But that was because my neighbor used to dump gasoline back there—and I didn't even have to pay a fine. They basically slapped my wrist." He also admits to stealing a cordless nail gun from an equipment rental store and, with his friends, running around for a week "blowing out car tires" until his parents found the nail gun and made him return it.

You ask more about the anger issue. He says he has road rage, and he will follow drivers who are foreign, especially Chinese, and try to get them to pull over so that he can "beat the shit out of them." He once tried to force the driver of a tractor-trailer to pull over because he thought the man had cut him off. He drives excessively fast and uses his headlights and car horn as he weaves through traffic. The feeling of rage comes over him instantly, and he feels he cannot stop it.

The anger also affects him in public places. Over the past 5 months, he has stayed at his mother's apartment as much as possible, mostly because he is afraid of starting fights. He started taking basic reading and writing classes at the community college, which he managed to attend sporadically, though he often left early or didn't show up at all because of this fear. He says he has no idea what people truly think about him, and he assumes the worst. He also says, "I really don't know who I am. This bothers me."

He tells you that he suffers extreme mood swings, and has since age 15. He describes two instances as a teenager when he felt his "engine run wild" for at least 10 days; his sleep decreased to 2–3 hours a night, and then he did not sleep for 3 days in a row. He felt euphoric during this time but denies having used drugs or alcohol. He remembers that he thought he could speak directly with God and that he was told he had a specific mission to bring happiness to his friends because the devil had found his family and was attempting to destroy them. He recalls being told by friends that it was difficult to understand what he was saying at the time, that his speech was "too fast" and "all over the place." There are gaps in his memory, periods when he does not remember exactly what he was doing, but he recalls that he "freaked out" his friends for a while. "They were afraid of me. I guess I got up into their faces about God even though I was never religious." He remembers being hypersexual during these times, cheating on a girlfriend with "at least three other girls, I don't know." He also started driving recklessly around the woods near his house, "doing doughnuts and trying to melt my tires, until the engine block cracked."

He says he started using drugs after the second such episode because it helped calm him down. After the second episode, he recalls his first extreme depressive episode where he felt suicidal. He lost interest in his friends for a time and became isolated; he did not leave his house except to go to school, but he did not talk to anyone there. He says, "It was weird; I just didn't care about anything anymore." He did not eat regularly and lost about 20 pounds in 2 months. His sleep was disturbed by frequent awakenings, during which he would feel the need to get up and pace around the house. "I just felt hopeless. I couldn't stop thinking about killing myself. I wasn't even doing drugs yet. That came later. I forced myself to meet a friend who got me high, and that seemed to help. I started going out more just to get high. But I was tired all the time. It took all my energy just to go out to get high with this dude, and I didn't even like him much."

He attempted suicide at age 16 by overdosing on his father's nitroglycerine tablets and drinking a pint of vodka. He has repeatedly had suicidal ideation, and he has a long history of self-mutilating behaviors that include slashing his wrists (although not with the intent to commit suicide), slashing his thighs, punching walls, and banging his head until it bleeds. He says that he is not currently suicidal and was not actually suicidal in the hospital; he had claimed he was in order to be admitted to the psychiatric inpatient unit because he felt that his anger was out of control.

His family had previously been more affluent. They lived in a lakefront house worth half a million dollars and had three boats, and his father bought him a brand-new truck for his 16th birthday. But 2 years ago his father sold the house because he had run up some $300,000 in debts, and a large portion of the proceeds of the house sale went to paying the debt. The patient has two brothers, one who has major depression that is being treated with an antidepressant. His mother also has bouts of depression and panic attacks, for which she takes an antidepressant and alprazolam; she has shared the alprazolam with the patient when he has been anxious and could not leave the house.

Until 5 months ago, he says, he was very outgoing, always had a girlfriend, had many other close friends (although they were drug users or dealers), and liked to go out to clubs. He has good relationships with his mother and his brothers. One of his brothers is homosexual, and the patient says this never bothered him, although he never completely understood why his brother turned out this way. His brother was accepted by his family when he "came out," and this was never an issue. The patient's "racism," which he describes primarily in terms of anger at Asians and Arabs, is very recent. He typically had friends from different cultural and racial backgrounds. However, he never kept any friends for more than 1 or 2 years. "They would do something to piss me off, I don't know. Then

I just blew them off. The same with my girlfriends. I wanted to marry my first girlfriend, but then I cheated on her."

Lately, since his father died, he has asked his mother to drive him back to the hospital where his father died so he can spit in the parking lot, find the doctor who treated him and punch him, or find the hospital vice president's car and slash the tires. He has even thought about killing himself by jumping off the hospital roof. Because of his overwhelming grief over his father's death and his often violent plans to "get back" at the doctors he believes were responsible, he and his mother have begun to fight more frequently, and she has threatened to kick him out of her house if he does not get help. They have stopped talking the way they used to, and he says he does not know how to talk to her anymore. He says he feels as if he is "about to snap" all the time, has difficulty concentrating and focusing, and is unable to read or even watch television without getting up and pacing, and his sleep is still disturbed with initial and middle insomnia.

DECISION POINT A

Given what you know about this patient, what is your differential diagnosis? (Multiple diagnoses are possible. +2 points for correct answers, −2 points for incorrect answers. Points also given for appropriate rule-outs, deducted for inappropriate rule-outs.)

Axis I:	
Axis II:	

DECISION POINT B

Create a problem list and name the five most relevant problems you would attempt to treat, in the order of their importance.

B1. _____ Alcohol abuse, anger management, major depression, social anxiety, insomnia

B2. _____ Alcohol abuse, suicidality and major depression, anger management, insomnia, grief

B3. _____ Alcohol abuse and cannabis dependence, mood instability, anger management, grief, anxiety

B4. _____ Alcohol abuse and cannabis dependence, anger management, mood instability, grief, anxiety

B5. _____ Grief, alcohol abuse and cannabis dependence, major depression, anger management, social anxiety

DECISION POINT C

Given what you know about the patient's diagnoses from Decision Point A, would you consider pharmacotherapy in addition to psychotherapy? If so, why? In what sequence? If not, why?

C1. _____ Once the patient has demonstrated sobriety for at least a month, his mood would be likely to

improve, and then he could engage more effectively in psychotherapy, which would be sufficient to manage the issues on his problem list.

C2. _____ Once the patient has demonstrated sobriety for at least a month, there is a chance that his mood would improve, although given his history of mood disorder as well as a family history of mood disorders, starting him on medication prior to psychotherapy would enable him to participate more fully.

C3. _____ Given the severity of this patient's mood disorder and his need for sobriety, he should be treated at the same time with drug and alcohol rehabilitation, cognitive behavior therapy, and psychopharmacotherapy.

C4. _____ Given the severity of this patient's mood disorder and his need for sobriety, he should be hospitalized until he is able to enter a partial hospitalization program in which he could receive a multidisciplinary approach to his many diagnoses.

C5. _____ You are not qualified to handle this patient. He has so many problems, so many diagnoses that are untreatable, that he should be transferred to a state hospital.

DECISION POINT D

The patient enters an outpatient substance abuse treatment program and starts attending AA meetings daily. He wants to work on his anger issue with you. What psychotherapy or psychotherapies would best address this problem?

D1. _____ Interpersonal psychotherapy
D2. _____ Dialectical behavior therapy
D3. _____ Cognitive behavior therapy
D4. _____ Supportive psychotherapy
D5. _____ Psychodynamic psychotherapy

DECISION POINT E

What are the four modules taught in dialectical behavior therapy?

E1. _____
E2. _____
E3. _____
E4. _____

ANSWERS: SCORING, RELATIVE WEIGHTS, AND COMMENTS

High positive scores (+3 and above) indicate a decision that would be effective and would be required for diagnosis, and without it, management would be negligent. Lower positive scores (+2) indicate a decision that is important but not immediately necessary. The lowest positive score (+1) indicates a decision that is potentially useful for diagnosis and treatment. A neutral score (0) indicates a decision that is neither clearly helpful nor harmful under the given circumstances. High negative scores (−5) indicate a decision that is inappropriate and potentially harmful or possibly life-threatening. Lower negative scores (−2 and above) indicate a decision that is nonproductive and potentially harmful.

DECISION POINT A

Axis I:	(+2) Bipolar I disorder, most recent episode depressed; (−2) rule out substance-induced mood disorder; (+2) alcohol abuse; (+2) cannabis dependence; (+2) rule out generalized anxiety disorder; (−2) rule out anxiety disorder not otherwise specified; (+2) rule out substance-induced anxiety disorder; (−2) rule out malingering; (−2) rule out adjustment disorder
Axis II:	(+2) rule out antisocial personality disorder; (+2) rule out histrionic personality disorder; (−2) border-line personality disorder

Axis I

Bipolar I disorder, most recent episode depressed: The patient describes at least two distinct episodes of mania as a teenager, including a distinct period of abnormally and persistently elevated and expansive mood lasting at least 1 week. During this time he felt as though he had a special mission, appointed by God, which represents grandiosity; he had a decreased need for sleep; he was reportedly hyperverbal and possibly pressured in speech; he had increased goal-directed activity; and he had excessive involvement in risky sexual behavior and reckless driving. The second episode was followed by major depression, during which he made a suicide attempt, was anhedonic, unintentionally lost weight, suffered insomnia, had feelings of hopelessness, had recurrent thoughts of death, and suffered daily fatigue. He has strong antisocial personality traits that by definition make it difficult to take his story at face value. Additionally, he comes from a dysfunctional family, and his father may have had bipolar disorder; there is a chance that much of his behavior is the result of having been spoiled and rich, with one experience at juvenile court that was dismissed, but otherwise few consequences as a teenaged boy. You might prefer to write "provisional" next to the diagnosis, since this patient's presentation and history

are so complicated that even with what seems to be a clear diagnosis of bipolar disorder, you are nevertheless unsure given his poor recollection. However, given his symptoms, treating him as if he has bipolar disorder would likely help him rather than hurt him.

His most recent episode is depressed.

Rule out substance-induced mood disorder: Despite the onset of bipolar I symptoms prior to his abuse of alcohol and drugs, it continued in the context of substance abuse. It is unlikely, however, given the more clear-cut diagnosis of bipolar I, that this mood disorder would have been diminished by the substance abuse. The latter is more likely a coping mechanism for the former.

Alcohol abuse: The patient engaged in a maladaptive pattern of drinking alcohol that worsened over a period of 6 months, including recurrent use despite the knowledge that it was hazardous and (given his driving under the influence) illegal, and continued use despite getting into fistfights, some of which were fueled by alcohol. He does not meet criteria for alcohol dependence.

Cannabis dependence: The patient developed tolerance to cannabis, used it in increasing amounts over several years, was unable to quit despite wanting to, spent a great deal of time obtaining the substance, felt that he had lost the desire "to do anything with my life," and continued using marijuana despite understanding that he was suffering physiological and psychological consequences (losing memory, amotivational syndrome).

Rule out generalized anxiety disorder: Given the concurrent use of substances and alcohol, it is difficult to make this diagnosis. However, the patient does express excessive anxiety and worry, especially since his father's death at least 6 months earlier. He is unable to control these symptoms and consequently drinks alcohol and uses drugs. He is excessively irritable, expresses an anger control problem and a desire to take revenge on the hospital and doctors where his father died, has difficulty concentrating, is "about to snap" all the time, and has a sleep disturbance. The stress is clinically significant, but it may be due to substance and alcohol abuse, which, although the criteria are clearly met for generalized anxiety disorder, does not satisfy the final diagnostic criterion, which is that the disturbance is not due to the direct physiological effects of a substance.

Rule out anxiety disorder not otherwise specified: The patient's symptoms meet the criteria for generalized anxiety disorder more fully.

Rule out substance-induced anxiety disorder: This is the alternative diagnosis to generalized anxiety disorder, given the patient's excessive drug and alcohol abuse. Although it seems that the patient developed these problems as a result of significant psychosocial stressors, the amount and frequency of his alcohol and substance abuse are significant. His symptoms prior to his father's death were more obviously bipolar I disorder, and he had no difficulty in social situations except during major depressive episodes.

Rule out malingering: The possibility that he is malingering is unlikely, as he is an alcohol abuser, is cannabis dependent, has strong antisocial traits stemming from a likely previous conduct disorder, and has current mood instability. These psychiatric conditions are not likely by intention for secondary gain. In this case, the secondary gain would be to stay out of jail for his DUI offense, as he assumes that he will be placed on probation. The patient was not referred by the courts or an attorney but by the hospital, and he came to you on his own for help. There is no discrepancy between his claimed stress or disability and objective findings. He is cooperative, and the likelihood of antisocial personality disorder is in the differential. These criteria suggest that malingering is unlikely.

Rule out adjustment disorder: This patient has had emotional and behavioral symptoms that were possibly exacerbated by identifiable stressors, such as the loss of his previous high standard of living and the loss of his father, but the stress-related disturbance better meets criteria for bipolar I disorder or any of the substance-induced mood disorders.

Axis II

It is too early to make a diagnosis of a personality disorder, especially in the context of a more obvious axis I diag-

nosis. Also, it is not in the patient's interest or helpful to the treating physicians to label him, for example, as having borderline personality disorder at this point, given the stigma that accompanies this diagnosis.

Rule out antisocial personality disorder: The patient does exhibit a pervasive pattern of disregard for and violation of the rights of others by his assaulting people, chasing other drivers on the highway, impulsivity, irritability and aggressiveness, reckless disregard for the safety of himself and others, and setting the woods on fire at age 14. He also engaged in reckless disregard for the property of others by stealing a nail gun and damaging the car tires of strangers.

Rule out borderline personality disorder: The patient has a pattern of unstable and intense interpersonal relationships, switching friends almost yearly, then "blowing them off" when they "piss him off." He reports that he does not know what people think of him and he does not understand himself, which suggests an identity disturbance. He has impulsivity as described above, involving sex, substance abuse, and reckless driving. He has had recurrent self-mutilating behaviors, affective instability, inappropriate, intense anger and difficulty controlling his anger, and some possibly stress-related paranoid ideation.

Rule out histrionic personality disorder: He has been inappropriately sexually seductive and provocative, cheating on his girlfriend, acting out hypersexuality; has rapidly shifting and shallow expression of emotions; and comes to his appointment dressed in a suit.

He does not exhibit substantial symptoms of narcissistic personality disorder.

Note: Many of these symptoms are confluent with bipolar disorder and the various substance-related disorders, so a diagnosis of a personality disorder is not necessarily accurate. The traits may exist or may have existed prior to the onset of the axis I disorder, such as setting the fire at age 14, which is suggestive of conduct disorder. However, since the picture is so complicated by the more clear diagnosis of bipolar disorder and the overwhelming influence of drug and alcohol abuse, these traits may represent exaggerations of personality styles.

DECISION POINT B

The purpose of this section is to help you consider how to approach a patient with such a complicated presentation, given all the treatment modalities in your armory. There are no perfect solutions, just some that may be more effective than others.

Although this patient's symptoms meet criteria that would categorically assign his problems into a more convenient array of DSM-IV-TR diagnoses, it is useful to think of the individual's problem list separately. After careful consideration of the patient's biological factors, psychosocial factors, and motivation as well as your resources, including the time you have to spend with him, you must somehow reach a working strategy for how best to help him. There will inherently be variability according to the practitioner's own experience with each of these issues or with combinations of these issues. There are regional differences in the way psychiatrists and therapists approach dual-diagnosis patients. Some advocate a harm reduction approach, whereas others insist on sequencing treatment (under the assumption that, for example, the depression cannot be addressed until the substance use is under control). There is no evidence that one strategy is significantly superior to another.

For example, whether to treat the drug and alcohol addictions before beginning treatment of any other issues is the standard of care for some clinicians, while treating both at the same time works well for others. The idea behind the former is that you cannot understand what the underlying psychiatric conditions are until you remove the confounding interference of mood-altering substances and alcohol. At that point, many would argue, the mood disorders or other symptoms might abate, rendering their treatment redundant.

However, others find that the reason for discriminating between diagnoses—and in fact calling them dual diagnoses—is that there are now two problems to treat, no matter which one came first. For the purposes of this particular exercise, there are multiple correct answers, although points are deducted for misdiagnoses. This patient has numerous issues that need treatment, and much more data must be gathered. Because of the nature of his potential diagnoses, the symptoms he admits to, the manner by which he presents, the possible undiagnosed conduct disorder as a teen and now the potential for antisocial personality disorder, and his needing you for legal purposes if he is on probation, you must be skeptical of everything he says.

B1. _____ −2 The patient meets criteria for cannabis dependence, not just alcohol abuse, so ignoring the other substance would possibly be dangerous to the patient.

B2. _____ −2 Again, the patient has cannabis dependence.

B3. _____ +2 Dealing with the alcohol abuse and cannabis dependence first is paramount in this patient; he absolutely must stay sober, both for his own physical and mental health and because of his probation. Even if you consider his history with skepticism because of the complications of the other diagnoses, you may consider that he meets criteria for bipolar I disorder and should be treated for that immediately, as his impulsiveness may be linked to this primary diagnosis. His anger management may become easier to treat, as it became a chief concern only recently, and it too may be linked to impulsivity and extreme fluctuations of mood related to psychosocial stressors, such as the dying and death of his father, with whom he was very close.

B4. _____ +1 Again, identifying and treating alcohol abuse and cannabis dependence is of paramount impor-

tance. Whether to work on his anger management first is the prerogative of the clinician. However, it is more likely that his anger issues have their origins in the bipolar disorder and perhaps his strong cluster B personality traits. He does need to deal with his grief, since his father died only recently and he has developed maladaptive coping strategies, which have manifested themselves in a possible generalized anxiety disorder.

B5. _____ +1 If grief, alcohol abuse, and cannabis dependence were treated at the same time, this order would make sense. The mood disorder should follow immediately, as it is likely the fuel for the anger and generalized anxiety issues.

DECISION POINT C

C1. _____ −2 This patient's alcohol abuse and cannabis dependence are a primary concern; however, his bipolar disorder preceded the use of alcohol and drugs, making this a clear diagnosis. He must be treated pharmacologically for bipolar disorder, especially given the severity of his symptoms. Psychotherapy can begin concurrently, but to neglect psychopharmacotherapy would not be helpful to this patient.

C2. _____ +2 It is a good idea to address the alcohol abuse and cannabis dependence as well as to follow this treatment with psychopharmacotherapy, but there is disagreement as to whether one should be done before the other or both at the same time. In this patient, the symptoms of his mood disorder and his alcohol abuse and cannabis dependence are so severe that beginning both treatments at the same time would likely yield more effective results more quickly.

C3. _____ +3 This is an example of a patient for whom all modalities of treatment could possibly and favorably be initiated concurrently, especially in dealing with the alcohol abuse and cannabis dependence, which themselves, if unchecked, would hinder the utility of beginning psychopharmacotherapy or psychotherapy for his bipolar disorder, anger issues, grief, and possible generalized anxiety disorder. A drawback of this approach would be that the patient is so unstable that he should be in a partial hospitalization program at the beginning of treatment to ensure that he is stabilized and able to address his issues without a crutch. See C4 for why this only receives +3 points.

C4. _____ +3 If the patient agrees, if there is adequate insurance to cover partial hospitalization, and if there is a partial hospitalization program available to this patient that would address all of his needs, this would be ideal. A drawback would be using partial institutionalization as a crutch for a patient who must learn to cope on his own if he truly wishes to make changes. See C3 for why this only receives +3 points.

C5. _____ −5 While this patient's problems seem insurmountable, you are a skilled psychiatrist with many options available to you. Giving up and sending the patient to a state hospital would not be in his best interest and would likely prove harmful to him. He needs to learn to take charge of his own problems, to adhere to a medication regimen, and to engage in psychotherapy if he truly wants to change. It may turn out that he is unable to do these things, but ample opportunities need to be offered before such a drastic step is taken.

DECISION POINT D

This patient's alcohol abuse and cannabis dependence must be addressed at the beginning. You will not be able to work on anything else with him until he is sober. Additionally, given your limited knowledge of his previous psychopharmacotherapy trials, you do not know enough to judge whether he will respond to a different agent, whether he did not have adequate trials of the medications he tried in the past, or whether his use of drugs and alcohol made any previous psychopharmacotherapy trials irrelevant.

With this patient, you have to build trust, develop a rapport, and establish a solid working therapeutic relationship, or else you will undoubtedly fail no matter what you try. He has been manipulative in the past and is very possibly being manipulative right now, since he needs to be involved in therapy for legal reasons; given his antisocial traits, you cannot completely trust what he says. You have to give him the impression that you respect him to a degree but that your respect has its limits. He must feel that he is working with you, not for you, and that he is not doing things just because you tell him to. Jumping straight into more structured cognitive behavior therapy-type exercises will be lost on him until he decides he can and wants to work with you. At that point, cognitive behavior therapy or dialectical behavior therapy would be excellent choices for working with his anger issues.

The following is a helpful way of summarizing the different psychotherapy modalities.

Dialectical behavior therapy: This is good therapy for just about anyone. However, it is especially suited to patients whose coping skills are damaged in very basic ways. It is also good for patients who do not have a great deal of insight. It entails learning how to feel, how to emote, how to react, how to trust, and how to cope with feelings with a larger palette of emotions and responses. The therapy includes homework in which newly learned skills and coping strategies are practiced.

A dialectic involves understanding the opposing perspectives of a thesis and an antithesis with the purpose of creating a synthesis that is more adaptive. In the case of dialectical behavior therapy, the thesis may be the "emotional mind," the way the patient feels. The antithesis is the "rational mind," or the facts surrounding the circumstances—often what the patient experiences as a crisis—that brought about the emotions. The synthesis represents the middle ground where the patient learns to use the emotions, combine them with his or her understanding of the facts, and develop a more adaptive strategy for thinking about the circumstances that brought on the crisis. Dialectical behavior therapy addresses the negative environment felt by the patient with careful, empathic validation techniques and helps the patient regulate his or her emotions, have more meaningful and understandable relationships with others, and tolerate the stressors that are inherent in the patient's world.

Cognitive behavior therapy: This therapy requires patient participation; homework is an important component. The patient may have to write things or try things. The patient should have some insight and the determination to make changes. Cognitive behavior therapy can be adaptable to many problems and is good for all types of patients. It may involve exposure and desensitization, techniques for addressing one's fears and anxieties, and then practicing greater mastery of them through more rational thoughts and behaviors. Cognitive behavior therapy can be seen as a supportive psychotherapy, supporting the ego. Mastery of anxiety and depression comes when the ego is strengthened to deal more effectively with situations previously perceived as dangerous—that is, as new skills are learned, the ego can better differentiate distortions. From a behavioral perspective, there is a delinking of affect from various situations so that, for example, by your 1,000th exposure to heights, you are not anxious about, but are now indifferent to, being on the 10th floor.

Interpersonal therapy: In this approach, depression is theorized to stem from one or more typical issues: a role transition, loss of a loved one, loss of a relationship. The issue is postulated to be the cause of the depression. It is a short-term therapy where the end is always in sight. It makes use of dynamic theories for the therapist, but no interpretations are offered as they would be in psychodynamic therapy.

Psychodynamic therapy: This approach requires higher-functioning patients who have good object relations, good superego function (a conscience), good impulse control, as well as the time and money for intensive psychotherapy. These patients do not require direct interventions. The therapy is directed toward understanding why they got to this particular place in their mental or emotional life; by understanding themselves better, they can move past it. Freud talked about making behavioral interventions with his agoraphobic patients in order for their dynamic therapy to proceed.

Supportive psychotherapy: This is psychotherapy that supports "ego function"—building up a patient's trust in you and in him- or herself, building ego strength, validating feelings, building a working alliance, and helping the patient through a difficult time with listening, advice, and validation. Much of it is "being there" for your patient.

There are techniques that are specific to supportive psychotherapy but that also spill over into many other forms of therapy. Thus, techniques such as clarification, encouragement, suggestion to elaborate, empathic validation, advice, and praise are used not only when doing supportive therapy but in doing all "higher" forms of therapy as well.

D1. ____ −2 Interpersonal psychotherapy. Not appropriate for anger management. This is for depression.

D2. ____ +3 Dialectical behavior therapy. Good therapy for this patient given the axis II issues.

D3. ____ +5 Cognitive behavior therapy. Especially good therapy for anger management.

D4. ____ +0 Supportive psychotherapy. As stated above, this patient requires supportive psychotherapy before he can address anything specific. But as a therapy to deal with anger management issues alone, this will not be sufficient.

D5. ____ +1 Psychodynamic psychotherapy. Making the interpretation at some point that the patient's anger around the loss of his father is being externalized, or that his sadness over the loss and his inability to do anything about it is frustrating to him, or that he is angry about the doctors who misdiagnosed his father's illness—which will come up in the transference between him and you as his current doctor—may prove beneficial, especially if he is able to internalize the interpretations and you are able to help make these gains permanent. However, given the acute nature of this patient's alcohol abuse and cannabis dependence and the dangerous nature of his impulsivity and violent tendencies, plus his limited insight at this time, this seems a less practical approach for now. In the future, after using a mixture of modalities, this may prove to be a highly effective treatment strategy.

DECISION POINT E

E1. ____ +2 **Mindfulness:** Using Psychological and behavioral versions of meditation practices from Eastern spiritual training, presented as three primary states of mind: "reasonable mind," "emotional mind," and "wise mind."

E2. ____ +2 **Interpersonal effectiveness:** Acquiring skills for obtaining changes one wants, maintaining the relationship, and maintaining self-respect. Includes developing the ability to analyze a situation and to determine goals.

E3. ____ +2 **Emotional regulation:** Addressing the struggles patients experience in regulating painful emotions that are central to behavioral difficulties.

E4. ____ +2 **Distress tolerance:** Learning how to accept, find meaning for, and tolerate distress.

KEY CLINICAL POINTS

1. In patients with a dual diagnosis, the standard of care for some clinicians is to treat drug and alcohol disorders first while other clinicians treat the dual diagnosis disorders concurrently.

2. The type of psychotherapy chosen is often based upon available resources and expertise. There are specific therapies that have been shown to be more effective than others for some disorders.

3. There are differences between short-term, structured psychotherapies, and longer-term insight-oriented psychotherapies. A psychiatrist should know which therapies are indicated as the most appropriate treatment.

YOUR TOTAL

Decision Point	Your Score	Ideal Best Score
A		14
B		4
C		8
D		9
E		8
Total		43

REFERENCES

American Psychiatric Association Practice Guidelines for the Treatment of Psychiatric Disorders, Compendium 2004, Washington, DC, American Psychiatric Publishing

Bachar E: Psychotherapy: an active agent: assessing the effectiveness of psychotherapy and its curative factors. Isr J Psychiatry Relat Sci 1998; 35:128–135

Dewald PA: Principles of supportive psychotherapy. Am J Psychother 1994; 48:505–518

Linehan M: Cognitive-Behavioral Treatment of Borderline Personality Disorder. New York, Guilford, 1993

Luborsky L: Theory and technique in dynamic psychotherapy: curative factors and training therapists to maximize them. Psychother Psychosom 1990; 53:50–57

Miller WR, Rollnick S: Motivational Interviewing: Preparing People for Change. New York, Guilford, 2002

Riba MB, Balon R: Competency in Combining Pharmacotherapy and Psychotherapy: Integrated and Split Treatment. Washington, DC, American Psychiatric Publishing, 2005

Rosenthal RN, Westreich L: Treatment of persons with dual diagnoses of substance use disorder and other psychological problems, in Addictions: A Comprehensive Guidebook. Edited by McCrady GA, Epstein EE. New York, Oxford University Press, 1999, pp 439–476

Sadock BJ, Sadock VA: Synopsis of Psychiatry, 10th ed. Philadelphia, Lippincott Williams & Wilkins, 2007

Weissman MM, Markowitz JC, Klerman GL: Comprehensive Guide to Interpersonal Psychotherapy. New York, Basic Books, 2000

Winston A, Rosenthal RN, Pinsker H: Introduction to Supportive Psychotherapy. Washington, DC, American Psychiatric Publishing, 2004

It's Like Squeezing
the End of a Garden Hose

VIGNETTE

You are an adult psychiatrist in private practice. A patient was referred to you by the local psychiatric emergency services for outpatient follow-up. He presented to the psychiatric emergency services six days earlier for feelings of worthlessness, helplessness, mild but persistent suicidal ideation without intention or plan, poor sleep with both initial and middle insomnia, waking 3–4 times per night. He says he has had insomnia since he was a teenager. He normally works out 6 times per week but has not been able to go to the gym for the past two months due to lack of energy and desire. He does not enjoy movies because he can't focus and says he typically would have gone to the theater once or twice per week. He is quite anxious, stating "my OCD is out of control." He tells you he has not lost or gained significant weight. After stabilization in the emergency room he contracted for safety and an appointment was set up for him to see you.

He arrives early for his appointment, dressed appropriately, well groomed, with good hygiene. You notice as he enters your office that he keeps his gaze fixed either to the floor or to you, but does not seem to notice his surroundings. He is friendly but does not offer his hand when you offer yours. He takes out a piece of tissue from the box beside the chair you offer and wipes the seat quickly before sitting down. He keeps his gaze fixed to yours.

You begin the interview. He is a 31-year-old single Asian-American male, currently unemployed, who moved back to your town approximately three months earlier to live with his father. He tells you he moved home to his father's house because he was having trouble while living with his mother in Korea. She and his father divorced when the patient was 17 years old. His mother returned to Korea while his father, who

is Caucasian, remained at home. He has a twin brother with whom he has not had any contact in nearly 10 years due to his brother's illness. "It's just impossible to deal with him," he tells you.

You ask what happened in Korea. He says he lived there for the past 1.5 years. He left Los Angeles, where he worked as a financial analyst for a major banking firm because he became addicted to injecting heroin and cocaine. He says he has been tested for HIV and hepatitis and is negative. He tells you he did share needles and purposely used dirty needles to try and die. He has many friends, some are highly educated professionals; they performed an intervention to get the patient to quit using drugs and get help. He went to an inpatient rehabilitation center in Los Angeles for 14 days and then left for Korea. He says he stayed clean from heroin and cocaine since then.

He remembers his mother thought he was a "fussy" baby. He remembers crying at the age of 5 years because his family lived in a house with a leaky faucet. He would cry when he heard the leaking faucet because he thought all of the world's water would drain away there unless it could be shut off. That's the first time he remembers checking faucets on a daily basis. At first he would do it before bed-time, but by the time he was in junior high school he was also checking door locks because he thought his family might be robbed. He remembers as a child twisting his neck in a circle when he saw a corner because he did not like sharp edges. He would make the circle with his eyes and tongue as well because it felt like smoothing out the edges and for a short while he would feel less anxious. But the feeling would inevitably return. When he sees words, especially when they are on a sign or posted on a bulletin board, he has to rearrange the letters into every conceivable pattern, then assigns numerical values for the letters and performs calculations multiplying each number by 2. If he does not do this in a particular order he has to start again.

He also started making grunting noises as a child and his parents took him to the pediatrician because they thought he had a respiratory illness. He has continued to make this sound until the present and he demonstrates for you. He says he also has to take a quick, deep guttural breath before pronouncing certain syllables in words. He sometimes can control these tics but he will have to let them loose later. "It's like squeezing the end of a garden hose," he explains. "Eventually, once I let go, it comes out in a torrent." He denies ever using foul language. He has uttered words like "pinball" or "simple", but has no explanation why these particular words. He tells you he started grunting and blurting out words before the age of 10. He moves his elbow in a circular motion, sticks out his tongue, and often touches any person standing near to him on the shoulder unconsciously. He finds he can stop these involuntary movements with great concentration and distraction, but inevitably once he relaxes or stops whatever activity was helping him "hold back" the tics, he will have a "tic explosion." He has been exhibiting these tics since he was 7 or 8 years old, he says.

Sometimes, he tells you, he has a panic attack. They are typically unprovoked, "out-of-the-blue", lasting 10–15 minutes, during which he feels diaphoretic, has chest pain and palpitations, and gets a feeling of impending doom. "Sometimes I think I'm about to die, like I'm having a heart attack or losing my mind." He has had episodes when he was afraid to go into public places because he feared he would have a panic attack or otherwise lose control of himself and have no way to escape. "It's horrible and embarrassing," he tells you. "Sometimes I just stay at home rather than risk it. Other times, however, I manage to forget about it and go out." The attacks began when he was a young boy, before he started using alcohol or drugs.

He tells you that he used alcohol, cocaine, heroin, marijuana, ecstasy, LSD, and prescription narcotics to try and relax or stop the tics and checking behaviors when they took over his days and kept him from work. When he uses the drugs he doesn't feel high but is able to stop the behaviors. However, the drugs eventually became a problem; they are difficult to obtain and he ran the risk of getting fired from various jobs if he ever was caught. In between bouts of alcohol dependence he would switch to "my cocktail" of shooting up heroin, cocaine, and smoking marijuana, which he did for at least two and a half years at the longest.

His problem with alcohol began when he was 15, drinking on weekends with friends. This escalated rapidly until he was drinking daily as a junior and senior at a local private high school. He laughs when he tells you he was elected class president both years. He managed to excel in school academically, and participated in wrestling and tennis. His mother came to his events but his father did not; he felt he

had no one to push him to be better. He was nationally ranked in both sports as a junior, but quit as a senior during his parents divorce. During his senior year, he drank, first on weekends, then during the week. He began to show up at wrestling practice drunk, was reprimanded, and quit. He says it takes more and more alcohol to get drunk and if he stops he begins to shake, become diaphoretic, feels his heart racing, and feels nausea.

He has tried several times to stop drinking on his own but only succeeded some of the times. Other times he required the assistance of an intervention by family and friends and rehabilitation.

He has been in rehabilitation twice, once when he was in high school, also after an intervention by friends and family. He managed to stay clean from alcohol for several years, but then would relapse. He bounced between alcohol and harder drugs, kicking one for the other. He smokes two packs of cigarettes per day. He began smoking at 18, smoking just one or two per day, but gradually increased over the years to two packs. He has tried to quit numerous times and continues despite knowing the damage cigarette smoking is doing to his body.

He was hospitalized twice for psychiatric reasons relating to suicide attempts. Both hospitalizations were after overdoses. On another occasion he was taken to the emergency room after cutting his wrists, but after he was stitched up he eloped. He reports multiple bouts of major depression since high school, with long periods of remission. He tells you the depressive symptoms were not related to alcohol or drug abuse, but he cannot say this for certain since he has been using alcohol and various substances for so much of his life. He believes the depressive symptoms are related to his inability to control his OCD and tics.

His current depressive symptoms have lasted at least one year, worsening for the past two to three months. He denies hearing voices or visual hallucinations, denies delusions of paranoia or persecution, but is concerned about how others perceive him. "I am acutely aware of my problems, my tics, my drinking and drug use," he tells you plainly. "I did not get angry each time my family and friends held an intervention. In fact, I was relieved."

Since graduating from college with degrees in mechanical engineering and political science, he has held five different jobs. He was always very strong in mathematics. He did not pursue graduate school; he was hired as an engineer and financial analyst for between 1–2 years before he would quit and move away because his symptoms were becoming too difficult to hide or manage. He made money, invested it well, and moved to Korea to teach English, learn Korean and Japanese, and be close to his mother, and away from troubles at home.

He stayed clean and sober for the first 6 months, but then began drinking again. "All they have in Korea is alcohol," he tells you. "It's extremely strong, but I ended up drinking about a liter or more a day before I left." He got into an alcohol-fueled fight with a taxi driver and wound up in jail just before leaving the country. He tells you he often got into fights while drinking. He would pick fights with random men in clubs, and one time he did get in trouble with the law.

When you ask if he has a partner or love interest, his expression turns flat. Then he laughs. "No," he says. "The longest was about 1 month."

DECISION POINT A

Given what you know from the above history, what is your differential diagnosis? +2 points are given for correct answers, −2 points for incorrect.

AXIS I:	
AXIS II:	

DECISION POINT B

Which of the following most accurately describes the initial pharmacological treatment for obsessive-compulsive disorder?

B1. _____ Olanzapine
B2. _____ Clomipramine with lithium augmentation
B3. _____ Clomipramine
B4. _____ Nortriptyline
B5. _____ There is no effective pharmacological treatment for OCD. Only behavioral therapy is effective.

DECISION POINT C

Tourette syndrome has been shown to be comorbid with OCD in 27% of cases. Given that the tics of the patient's Tourette syndrome and OCD are negatively impacting his ability to function socially and at work, what pharmacologic strategy or strategies would best control his symptoms?

C1. _____ Paroxetine
C2. _____ Paroxetine and haloperidol
C3. _____ Paroxetine and fluphenazine
C4. _____ Methylphenidate
C5. _____ Clonidine

DECISION POINT D

Match the following medications used to treat alcoholism with their respective utility profiles:

Medication	Utility Profile
D1. Naltrexone	A. Protective against Wernicke's encephalopathy
D2. Acamprosate	B. Causes nausea when alcohol is consumed
D3. Nalmefene	C. Pure opioid receptor antagonist blunts pleasurable effects, reduces craving.
D4. Disulfiram	D. Thrice daily dosing, major side effect is diarrhea
D5. Thiamine	E. Pure opioid receptor antagonist blunts pleasurable effects, reduces craving, known for absence of dose-dependent liver toxicity and more effective binding to central opiate receptors.

Decision Point E

Given this patient's presentation, what medication(s) would you choose to treat his Panic Disorder with Agoraphobia? Rank the following medications by the order you would use them. Write "O" if you would not use them:

E1. _____ Clomipramine

E2. _____ Phenelzine

E3. _____ Paroxetine

E4. _____ Buspirone

E5. _____ Clonazepam

E6. _____ Alprazolam

Decision Point A

AXIS I:	(+2) Major Depressive Disorder, Recurrent, Severe, Without Psychotic Symptoms;
	(+2) Rule out Substance-Induced Mood Disorder;
	(+2) Obsessive Compulsive Disorder;
	(+2) Tourette Syndrome;
	(+2) Panic Disorder With Agoraphobia;
	(+2) Alcohol Dependence;
	(+2) Nicotine Dependence;
	(+2) Opiate Dependence in Sustained Full Remission;
	(+2) Cannabis Dependence in Sustained Full Remission;
	(+2) Cocaine Dependence in Sustained Full Remission;
	(+2) Polysubstance Dependence in Sustained Full Remission;
	(+2) Hallucinogen Abuse in Sustained Full Remission
AXIS II:	

Major depressive disorder, recurrent, severe, without psychotic symptoms: The patient complains of multiple episodes of major depression with intervals greater than 2 months between them. He complains of both depressed mood and anhedonia, and neither is due to a medical condition. Additionally he complains of depressed mood most of the day, diminished interest in activities, insomnia, loss of energy, feelings of worthlessness, poor concentration, and recurrent suicidal ideation. It is possible that these symptoms could be related to his extensive alcohol and drug use, but from the limited history it is not clear enough to make a definitive diagnosis of substance-induced mood disorder. For that reason, a rule-out for the latter diagnosis is appropriate. He does not complain of psychotic symptoms.

Obsessive-compulsive disorder: The patient complains of both obsessions and compulsions, including intrusive thoughts about cleanliness, sharp corners, the order of numbers. Many of these thoughts are seemingly arbitrary, not related to reallife problems. He attempts to avoid the thoughts about sharp edges and corners by averting his gaze when he comes into your office. He tells you about how he attempts to control the obsessive thoughts in certain social and occupational situations. He also has insight into the obsessive thoughts as products of his own mind. He compulsively washes, orders, checks, rearranges numbers, all to reduce the anxiety produced by the obsessive thoughts. He tells you these thoughts are "out of control" and recognizes these obsessions and compulsions have caused him to leave jobs

over the years. They cause marked distress, interfering with his normal occupational and social functioning, and are not restricted to a certain concern.

While it is possible these behaviors and thoughts are exacerbated by alcohol and substances, he reported that the first obsessive thoughts began when he was 5 years old.

Tourette's disorder: The patient had both multiple motor and one or more vocal tics that were present at some time during the illness. They occurred many times a day nearly every day or intermittently throughout a period of more than 1 year, and during this period there was never a tic-free period of more than 3 consecutive months. Onset was when the patient was 7 or 8 years old.

While it is possible that alcohol or substances may have exacerbated his symptoms, they occurred long before he began using.

Panic disorder with agoraphobia: The patient complains of recurrent, unexpected panic attacks that are followed by one month or more of persistent concern about having additional attacks, feeling like the patient is losing control, having a heart attack, or "losing my mind", and a significant change in behavior related to the attacks. The patient also complains of avoiding situations which might provoke the panic and stays at home.

Alcohol dependence: The patient has been drinking since he was a teenager with several periods of sobriety, but he is currently dependent. He demonstrates a maladaptive pattern of use manifest by tolerance, withdrawal syndrome, using larger quantities of the alcohol to achieve the desired affect, persistent efforts to cut down or quit, and has dropped or quit activities, such as wrestling, due to the alcohol dependence. He was arrested for starting fights while intoxicated and knows his problems worsen with the use of alcohol.

Nicotine dependence: The patient started with 1–2 cigarettes per day and eventually smoked 2 packs per day. He has tried unsuccessfully to cut down, suggesting withdrawal effects, and knows it is dangerous to him physically.

Opiate dependence in sustained full remission: The patient has not met criteria for dependence or abuse during a period of 12 months or longer.

Cannabis dependence in sustained full remission: The patient has not met criteria for dependence or abuse during a period of 12 months or longer.

Cocaine dependence in sustained full remission: The patient has not met criteria for dependence or abuse during a period of 12 months or longer.

Hallucinogen abuse in sustained full remission: The patient abused LSD and Ecstasy to help him cope with his OCD symptoms. He used them recurrently when he knew they would cause him to get fired from jobs. However, he has not used them for more than 12 months.

Polysubstance dependence in sustained full remission: The patient did use at least three different groups of substances not including caffeine and nicotine and he says that he would shift from alcohol to these other substances, suggesting one was not predominant (his "cocktail"). Dependence criteria were met for the substances individually, however, not only as a group. Additionally, he was in sustained remission from most of the substances. Therefore, although he meets criteria for polysubstance dependence in sustained full remission, it is also accurate in this case to list each substance and alcohol separately. This also helps the clinician to understand exactly what substance and alcohol problems the patient has or had.

−2 Obsessive-compulsive personality disorder: This diagnosis is for patients who demonstrate a preoccupation with orderliness, perfectionism, and mental and interpersonal control, at the expense of flexibility, openness, and efficiency, beginning by early adulthood and present in a variety of contexts, as indicated by four of eight criteria. This patient has more clear-cut obsessions and compulsions that are less well described as a personality or characterological style and more of an anxiety disorder.

DECISION POINT B

B1. _____ −3 The question asks for the most common initial treatment option. Since approximately 40% of OCD patients do not respond to SSRIs, olanzapine, an atypical antipsychotic, may be used alone or as an augmentation strategy if a patient does not improve on an SSRI or clomipramine. Also since patients are typically on anti-obsessional medications for long periods of time, you would have concerns about using danzapine initially given the risks of initiating a metabolic syndrome.

B2. _____ −2 This is a potent augmentation strategy especially for depression, however the question asks for the most common initial treatment option.

B3. _____ +5 The tricyclic antidepressant clomipramine is a potent serotonin reuptake inhibitor and the anti-OCD effect has been linked to this property. The neurotransmitter(s) correlated with OCD have not been conclusively identified, and it is likely there are more than one involved; the serotonin hypothesis still dominates the logic behind the treatment of OCD. The evidence of comorbid depression with OCD supports the utility of a serotonin reuptake blockade, although given the poor response of norepinephrine to treating the OCD suggests it is more sensitive to the serotonin reuptake blockade. Additionally, treatment of the OCD takes 12–26 weeks for a response, compared to 3–6 weeks for the relief of depressive symptoms. A substantial role for the neurotransmitter dopamine is suggested by the relationship between OCD symptoms and certain neurological disorders that feature seemingly purposeless, complex, repetitive behaviors as found in OCD. Additionally, chronic motor tic symptoms featuring the dysfunction of dopamine in the basal ganglia such as Von Economo encephalitis, Tourette syndrome, and Sydenham chorea, suggest a substantial role for this neurotransmitter. Subsequently, many patients do not respond well with an SSRI monotherapy and a variety of augmentation strategies may be tried.

B4. _____ −3 There is no strong evidence that a norepinephrine reuptake blockade is effective in anti-OCD action. Trials using noradrenergic reuptake inhibitors such as nortriptyline or desipramine have little to no anti-OCD action.

B5. _____ −5 Behavioral therapy is the most common adjunct therapy to pharmacotherapy. However, it is as effective in the treatment of OCD in selected cases and is often employed before the use of pharmacotherapy. This question, however, asks specifically for the correct medication.

DECISION POINT C

C1. _____ +3 Since 45 to 90% of Tourette syndrome patients have a history of comorbid OCD, the use of an SSRI is a reasonable first choice.

C2. _____ +5 The use of an SSRI is appropriate for treating the OCD, while a dopamine receptor antagonist is effective at controlling tics. Traditionally, older antipsychotics such as fluphenazine and pimozide are employed for this purpose. These typical have been shown to be more effective and better tolerated than haloperidol.

C3. _____ +5 See above.

C4. _____ −3 Although it was previously felt that a stimulant would cause or worsen tics, one study of 136 children with comorbid ADHD and Tourette syndrome demonstrated a lessening of tic severity compared to placebo, a similar number of patients with worsening tics comparing methylphenidate, clonidine plus methylphenidate, and placebo (20, 26, and 22% respectively). However, using a stimulant in a patient whose only symptom is tics has not been demonstrated as effective.

C5. _____ +3 This medication is more effective with comorbid Tourette syndrome and predominant behavioral, impulse control, and rage control symptoms. While this patient has experienced rage control episodes, has poor impulse control, his OCD is predominantly of the classic variety.

DECISION POINT D

This question emphasizes the pharmacotherapies for the treatment of alcoholism. It is well-established that group, especially peer-group therapies, with or without medication is most effective.

D1. _____ +2 C Naltrexone is a pure opioid receptor antagonist that blunts the pleasurable effects of alcohol and reduces craving. The number of drinking days is reduced as is relapse. It is felt to improve resistance to thoughts about drinking. However, relapse after discontinuation of naltrexone is common. The most common side effects are headache, arthalgias, anxiety and sedation. Naltrexone can cause hepatocellular injury and subsequently should not be given to patients with acute hepatitis or liver failure. Prior to initiating treatment, liver function tests should be performed.

D2. _____ +2 D Acamprosate decreases excitatory glutamergic neurotransmission during alcohol withdrawal and thus was approved for relapse prevention. Guidelines suggest starting acamprosate as soon as possible after abstinence with thrice daily dosing. Some suggest the thrice daily dosing is appealing to this population because they are psychologically used to regular maintenance of their alcohol dependence, thus increasing likelihood of compliance. The major side effect is diarrhea.

D3. _____ +2 E Nalmefene is a newer opioid receptor antagonist that does not have dose-dependent liver toxicity as with naltrexone, and more effective binding to central opiate receptors.

It has not yet been approved for use for alcohol abuse by the FDA.

D4. _____ +2 B Disulfiram, inhibits activity of acetaldehyde dehydrogenase (ALDH). The ingestion of alcohol causes increased plasma levels of acetaldehyde, leading to facial flushing, tachycardia, hypotension, dyspnea, nausea, vomiting, headache, blurred vision, vertigo, and anxiety within 15–30 minutes, lasting several hours. The inhibitory activity lasts for several days. Dangers associated with disulfiram include violent reactions to anything containing alcohol, such as cough syrups or sauces. It can cause hepatotoxicity, increases drug levels of phenytoin, isoniazid, and anticoagulants. It can cause hepatitis.

D5. _____ +2 A Thiamine is a cofactor for several key enzymes important in energy metabolism, including transketolase, alphaketoglutarate dehydrogenase, and pyruvate dehydrogenase. In alcoholics, thiamine deficiency is typically caused by inadequate dietary intake, reduced gastrointestinal absorption, decreased hepatic storage, and impaired utilization. The etiology of the thiamine-deficiency brain lesions is unclear, however studies have linked this deficiency with Wernicke's encephalopathy, described first in 1881 by Carle Wernicke, as mental confusion, ophthalmoplegia, and gait ataxia.

DECISION POINT E

SSRIs, tricyclics, benzodiazepines, and MAOIs have all been shown to be effective treatments for Panic Disorder when compared to placebo. The primary differences for choosing between them are related to their side effect profiles. SSRIs are first-line choices because of their safety and relatively low side effects when compared to the other choices. However, since they often cause symptoms of jitteriness, agitation, restlessness, headache, insomnia, gastrointestinal problems such as diarrhea or nausea, recommended starting doses are low followed by slow titration to the optimal effective dose. The response time is typically 4–6 weeks, and if there is no response by 8–12 weeks, another class could be tried.

Tricyclics are less expensive, but anticholinergic properties and sedation are often cited as reasons for trying an SSRI first. However, if a patient has had good experience with tricyclics, they may be used as a first line treatment. Imipramine and clomipramine are the most well-studied of the group. Nortriptyline is better tolerated than imipramine and clomipramine.

Benzodiazepines have been demonstrated to be effective for patients who are unable to tolerate or do not respond favorably to antidepressants. Using longer-life benzodiazepines such as clonazepam are less likely to cause the rebound anxiety that is often experienced by using shorter half-life benzodiazepines. Because of the highly addictive nature of this class of medication, use in patients with comorbid substance or alcohol abuse is not advised. Combination treatment with an SSRI, slowly tapering the benzodiazepine as the SSRI becomes effective has shown to be effective.

MAOIs are considered as effective as the other medications mentioned, however they are infrequently used because of orthostatic hypotension, the tyramine-free diet restriction, numerous dangerous drug-drug interactions, and other intolerable side effects. EMSAM, a transdermal patch form of selegeline, was approved by the FDA in 2006 for use in the treatment of depression. By bypassing the gut, the need for a tyramine diet is not necessary. As of this writing there have not yet been any studies of the transdermal form of selegeline for panic disorder. Given the more favorable side effect profile, however, clinicians may choose such an MAOI more readily.

Buspirone is used as an anxiolytic but has not been demonstrated to be effective in the treatment of panic disorder.

E1. 2   +2
E2. 3   +2
E3. 1   +2
E4. 0   +2
E5. 2   +2
E6. 2   +2

The reader should keep in mind that the above presentation is of an individual with numerous psychiatric diagnoses derived from unclear etiologies. In all likelihood such a patient would require a multidisciplinary approach to his many issues and a combination of medications which would likely require a fair measure of trial and error. For the purposes of this exercise, the reader should bear in mind there are also differences across the country regarding the treatment of dual diagnosis patients, differences in insurance formularies dictating the availability of some of these medications, differences in socio-economic status or access to adequate mental health care.

YOUR TOTAL

Decision Point	Your Score	Ideal Best Score
A		24
B		5
C		16
D		10
E		12
Total		67

KEY CLINICAL POINTS

1. In creating the differential diagnosis it is important to understand the co-morbidities of substance abuse and dependence and underlying psychiatric disorders.
2. Naltrexone, acamprosate, and disulfiram, medications used to treat alcoholism have different utility profiles.
3. Clomipramine, fluoxetine, fluvoxamine, paroxetine, and sertraline, are pharmacological agents used for the treatment of OCD. In choosing among the SSRIs, the psychiatrist should consider safety and side effects for the patient, including any applicable FDA warnings, potential drug interactions, past treatment response, and the presence of co-occurring general medical conditions.

REFERENCES

Acamprosate campral for alcoholism. Med Lett Drugs Ther 2005; 47:1

American Psychiatric Association Practice Guidelines for the Treatment of Psychiatric Disorders, Compendium 2004, Washington, DC, American Psychiatric Publishing, 2004

Ballenger, JC, Wheadon, DE, Steiner, M, et al. Double-blind, fixed-dose, placebo-controlled study of paroxetine in the treatment of panic disorder. Am J Psychiatry 1998; 155:36

Black, DW, Wesner, R, Bowers, W, Gabel, J. A comparison of fluvoxamine, cognitive therapy, and placebo in the treatment of panic disorder. Arch Gen Psychiatry 1993; 50:44

Freeman, RD, Fast, DK, Burd, L, et al. An international perspective on Tourette syndrome: selected findings from 3,500 individuals in 22 countries. Dev Med Child Neurol 2000; 42:436.Kenney, C, Jankovic, J. Tetrabenazine in the treatment of hyperkinetic movement disorders. Expert Rev Neurother 2006; 6:7

Lydiard, RB. Panic disorder: Pharmacologic treatment. Psychiatr Ann 1988; 18:468

Lydiard, RB. Drug treatment of panic disorder. In: Hypnotics and anxiolytics, Nutt, DG, Mendelson, WB (Eds), Ballierre Tindall, London 1995. p.427

Mason, BJ, Ritvo, EC, Morgan, RO, et al. A double-blind, placebo-controlled pilot study to evaluate the efficacy and safety of oral nalmefene HCl for alcohol dependence. Alcohol Clin Exp Res 1994; 18:1162

Nass, R, Bressman, S. Attention deficit hyperactivity disorder and Tourette syndrome: what's the best treatment?. Neurology 2002; 58:513

Otto, MW, Tuby, KS, Gould, RA, et al. An effect-size analysis of the relative efficacy and tolerability of serotonin selective reuptake inhibitors for panic disorder. Am J Psychiatry 2001; 158:1989

Piacentini, J, Chang, S. Behavioral treatments for Tourette syndrome and tic disorders: state of the art. Adv Neurol 2001; 85:319

Roy-Byrne, PP, Katon, W. An update on treatment of the anxiety disorders. Hosp Community Psychiatry 1987; 38:835

Silay, YS, Jankovic, J. Emerging drugs in Tourette syndrome. Expert Opin Emerg Drugs 2005; 10:365

Stahl SM, Essential Psychopharmacology, Second Edition. New York: Cambridge University Press, 2000

Treatment of ADHD in children with tics: a randomized controlled trial. Neurology 2002; 58:527

Volpicelli, JR, Volpicelli, LA, O'Brien, CP. Medical management of alcohol dependence: Clinical use and limitations of naltrexone treatment. Alcohol Alcohol 1995; 30:789